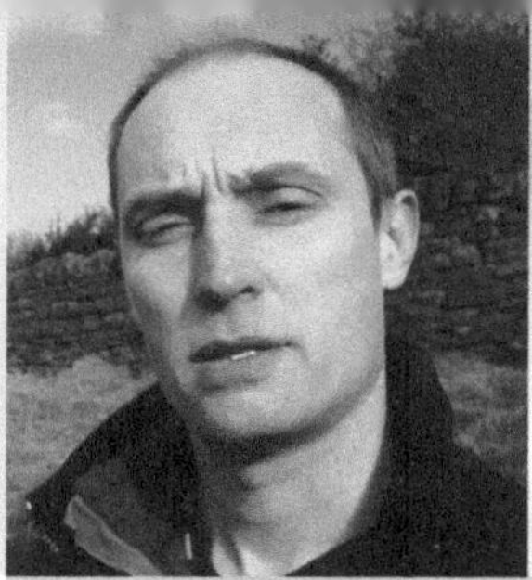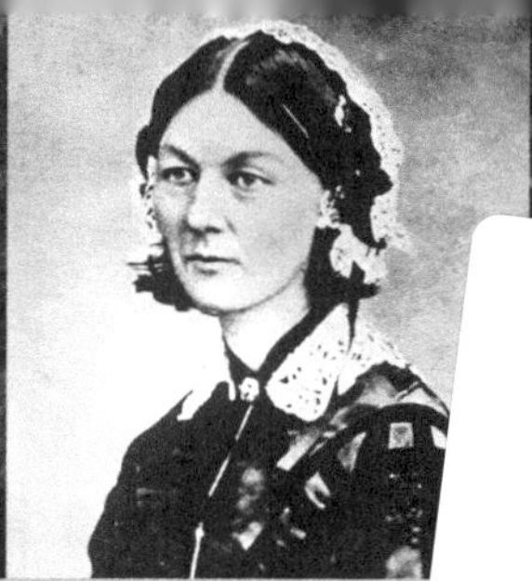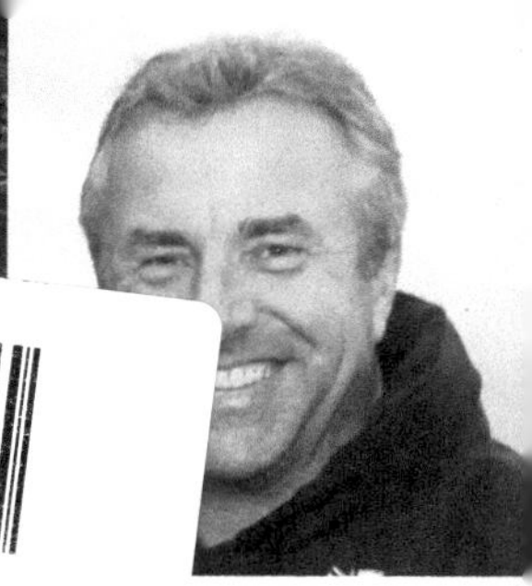

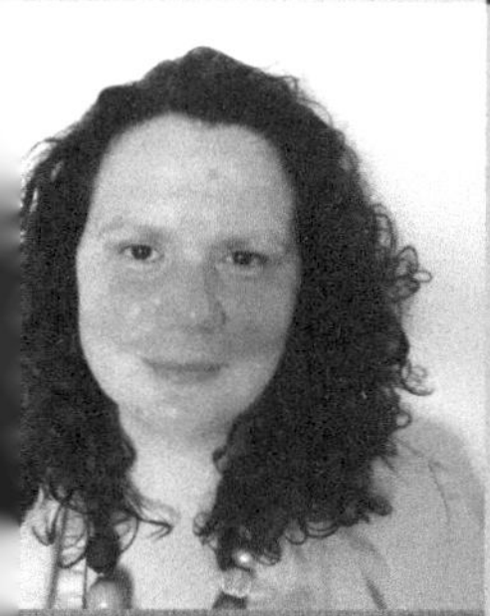

Mental Health Recovery Heroes Past and Present

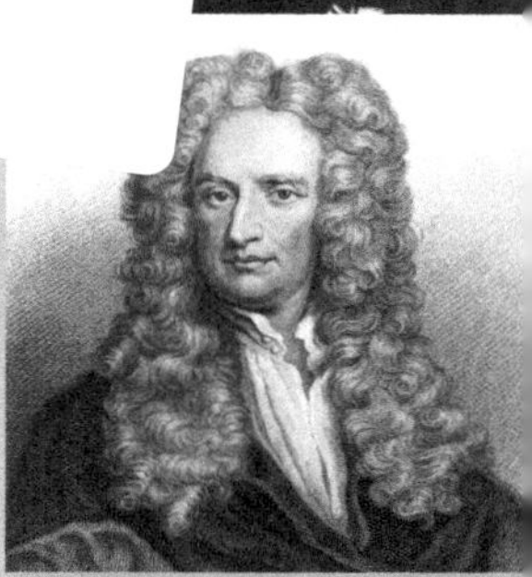

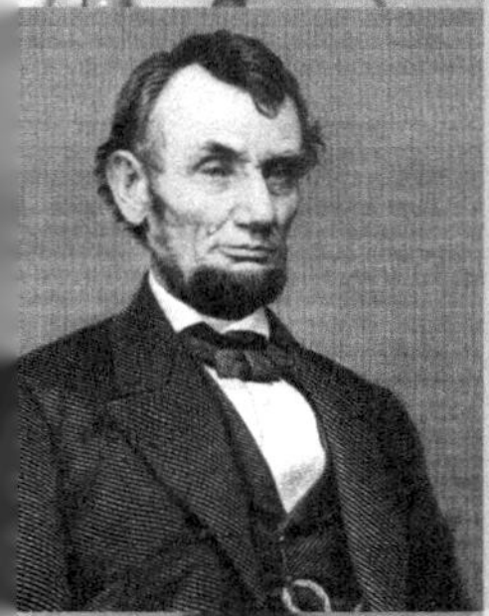

A handbook for mental health care staff, service users and carers

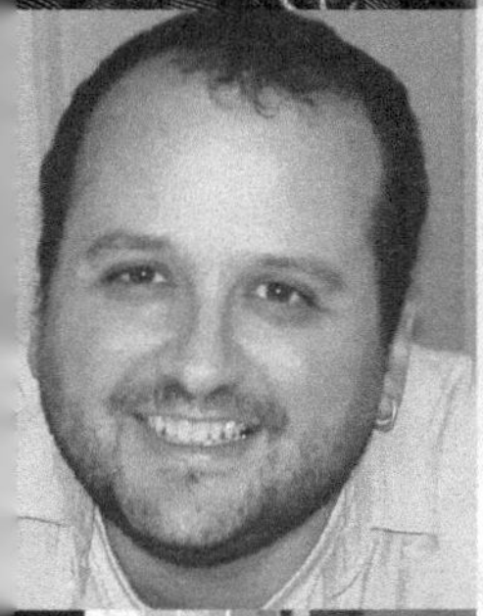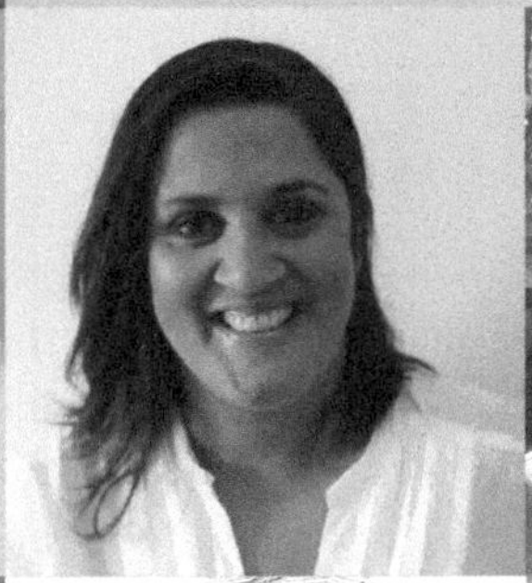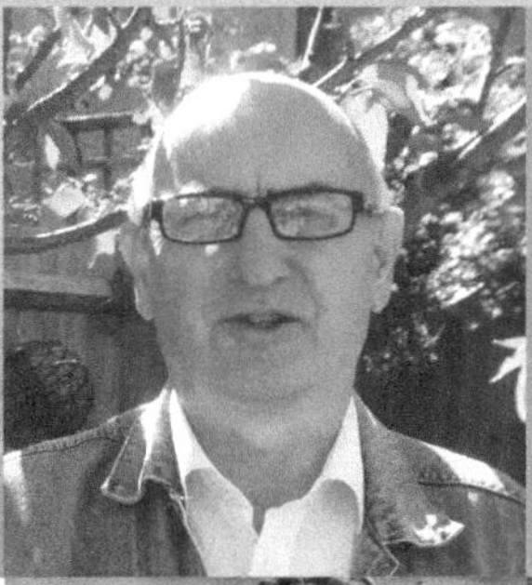

Sophie Davies, Elizabeth Wakely, Sarah Morgan and Jerome Carson

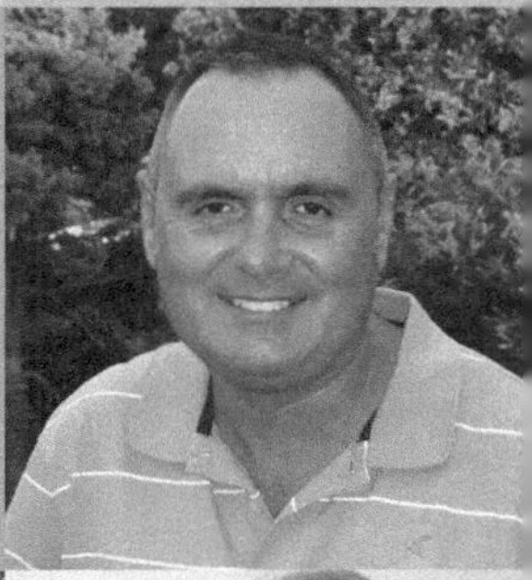

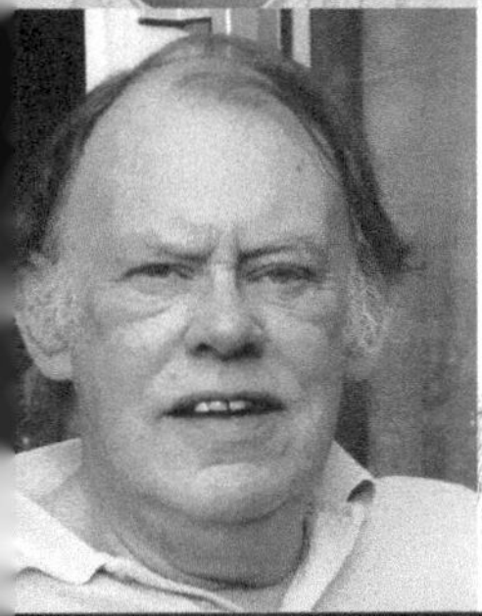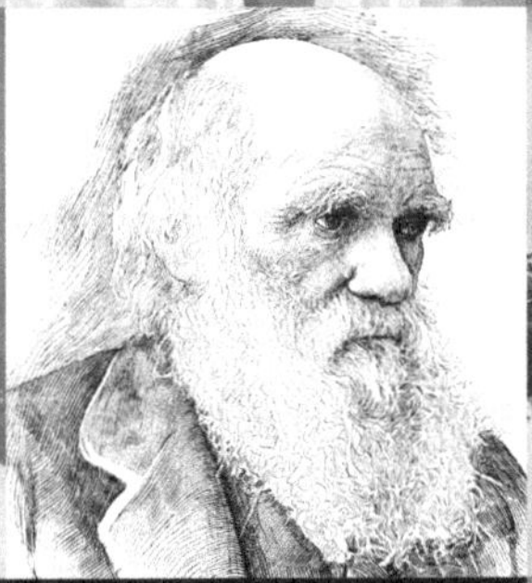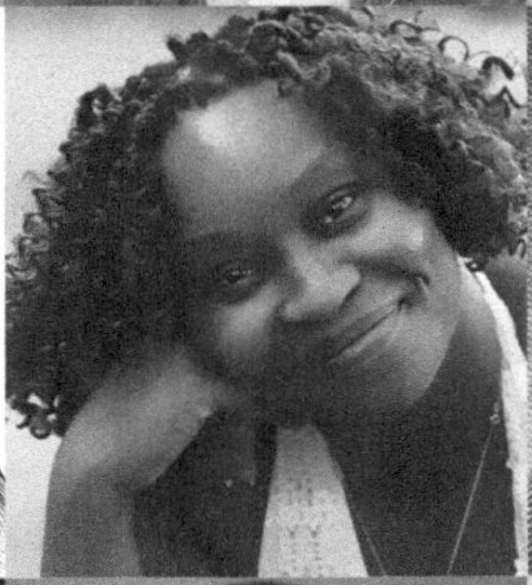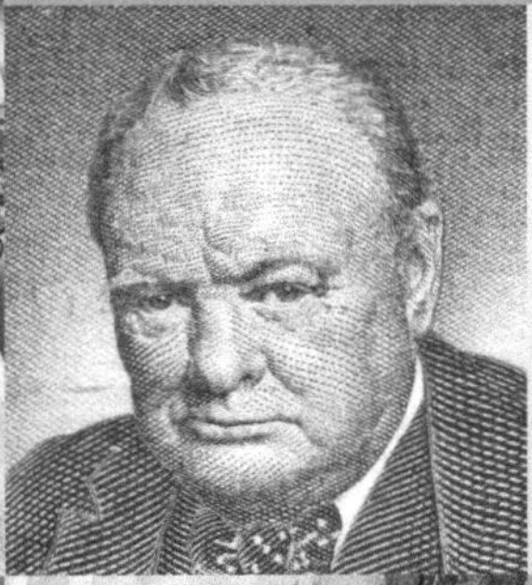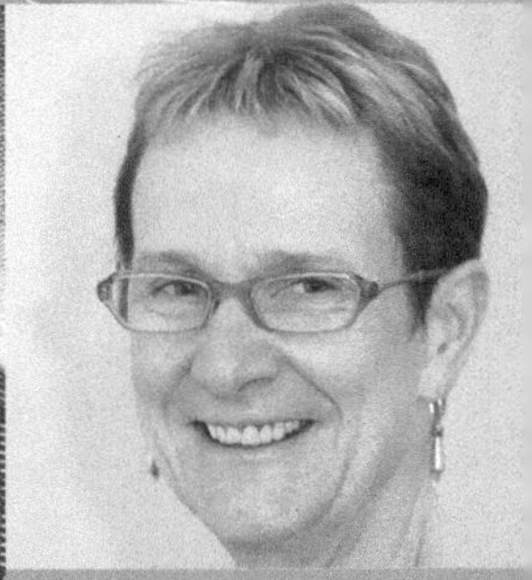

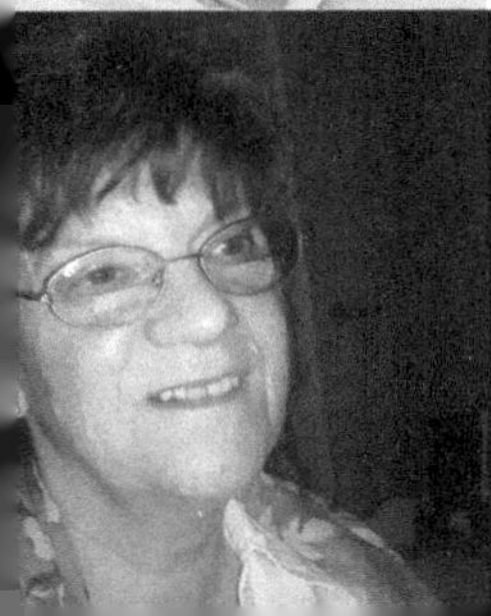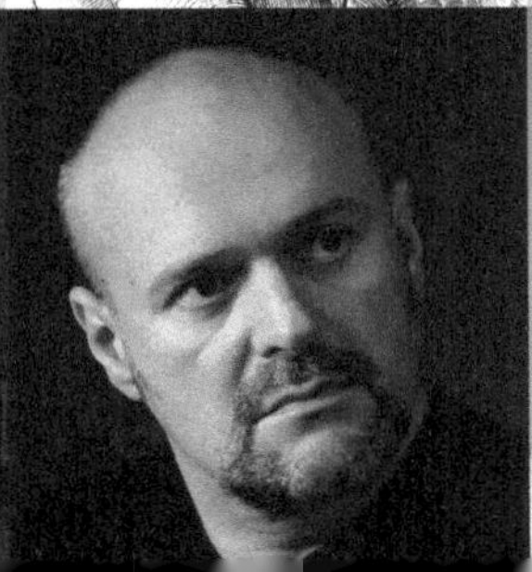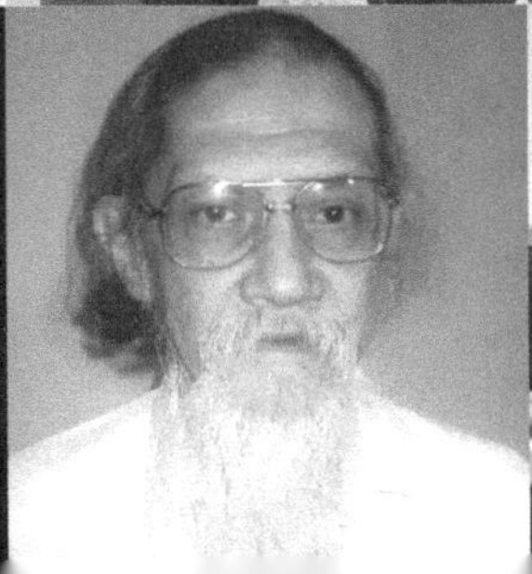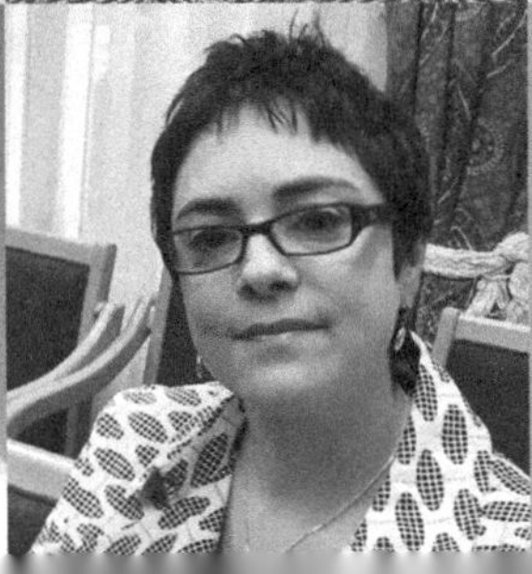

Pavilion

Mental Health Recovery Heroes Past and Present

A handbook for mental health care staff, service users and carers

Published by:
Pavilion Publishing and Media Ltd
Rayford House
School Road
Hove
BN3 5HX
UK

Tel: 01273 43 49 43
Fax: 01273 22 73 08
Email: info@pavpub.com
Web: www.pavpub.com

First published 2011, 2013

A Catalogue reference for this book is available from the British Library.

ISBN: 978-1-908066-54-1

Pavilion is the leading training and development provider and publisher in the health, social care and allied fields, providing a range of innovative training solutions underpinned by sound research and professional values. We aim to put our customers first, through excellent customer service and good value.

Editor: Sanaz Nazemi, Pavilion
Cover design and page layout: Tony Pitt, Pavilion
Typesetting: Emma Garbutt, Pavilion
Printed on paper from a sustainable resource by: Ashford Press

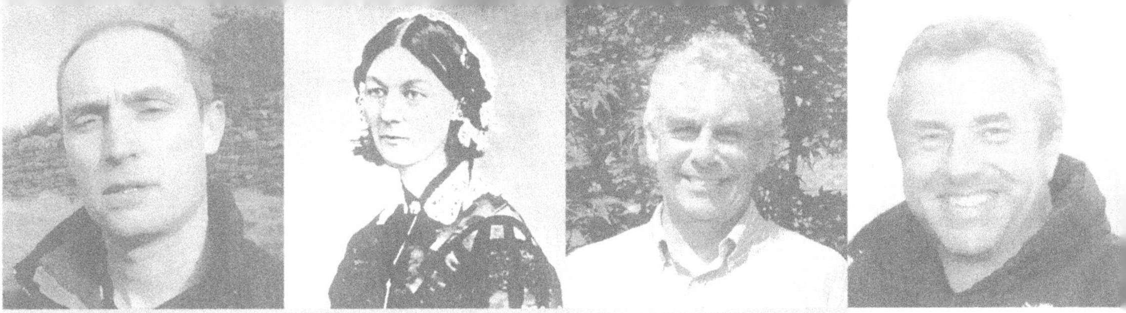

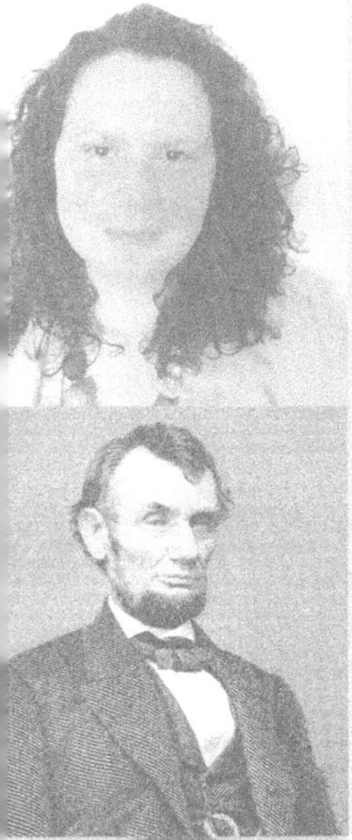

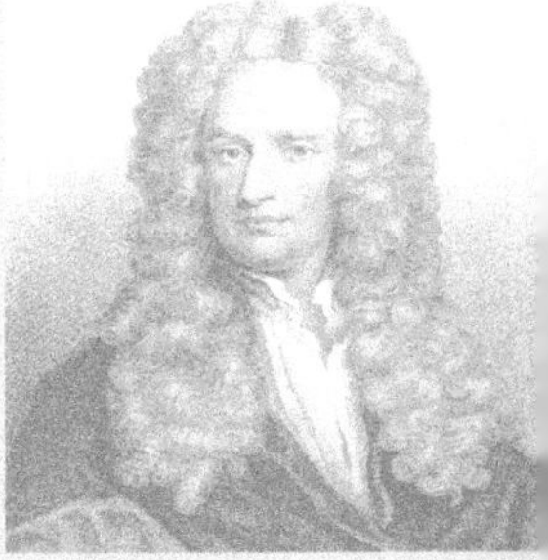

Mental Health Recovery Heroes Past and Present

A handbook for mental health care staff, service users and carers

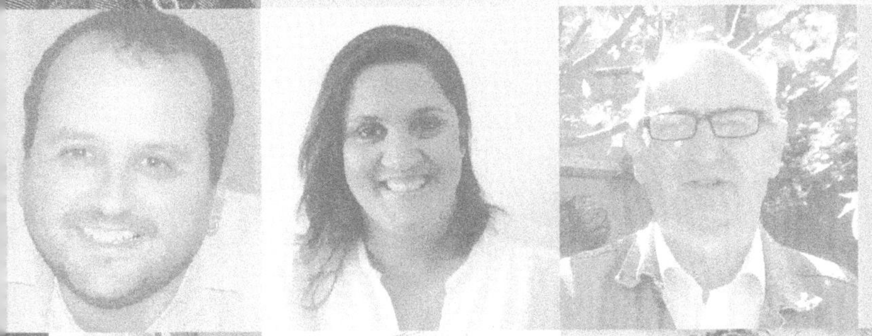

Sophie Davies, Elizabeth Wakely, Sarah Morgan and Jerome Carson

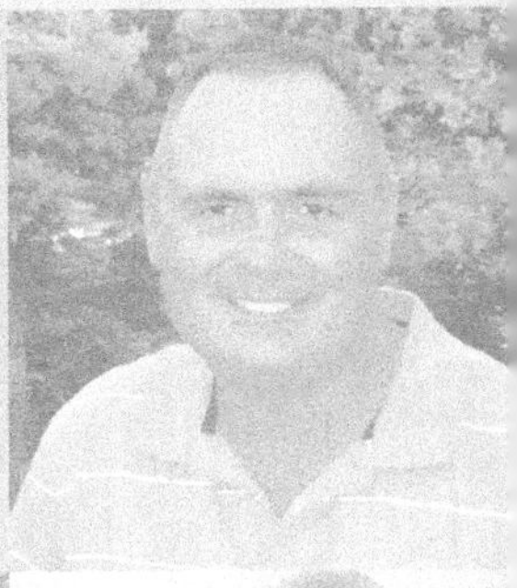

Pavilion

To Zeynab,
All the best for your future career in Psychology,

Contents

Foreword

Geoff Shepherd
Recovery Programme Lead, Centre for Mental Health, and visiting Professor for the Department of Health Services and Population Research, Institute of Psychiatry, University of London

This is a remarkable book. It deserves to reach the widest possible audience: mental health professionals – both qualified and in training – managers, commissioners, policy makers, service users and carers. There is truly something in here for everybody. I read it mainly as a professional, also as a researcher, and someone interested in improving the quality of mental health services.

The first thing to say is that, perhaps surprisingly, some of the contributors are rather sceptical about 'recovery'. Peter Bullimore says in Chapter 17, '*To be honest, I don't get that involved ... in recovery, because I think it's wrong when we are telling people how to recover ... what we need is love, compassion and guidance, we don't need tools for recovery, we don't need models for recovery ... we're turning recovery into a science, it has been hijacked by the services*'. This expresses a common worry for many people with mental health problems regarding recovery, but the book provides a strong counter argument. It is a simple, unadorned set of accounts of people's lives and is full of '*love, compassion and guidance*'. It does not contain a set of 'tools for recovery' or a 'model' (although a model could be drawn out of these rich and wonderful narratives). Thus, hopefully, Peter (and people like him) will forgive the authors for wanting to make his story and many others available to an audience who might otherwise never hear them.

Similarly, a number of the contributors are sceptical about the idea of 'recovery heroes'. '*I believe all who suffer the pain and anguish of mental illness are heroes*' (Margaret Muir, Chapter 9). '*I am not a recovery hero. It sounds a nice title to have and the other individuals in this series are all worthy of that title, but I am not. I am a recovery survivor*' (Matthew Ward, Chapter 14). I have to admit I was rather in agreement with Margaret and Matthew. In the introduction the authors make a distinction between the word 'hero' used in the Greek sense – '*individuals who, in the face of danger and adversity, showed either courage or self-sacrifice, for some greater good of all humanity*' – and 'hero' used in the 'routine' sense – individuals who struggle to find meaning and purpose in their lives and '*whose journey of recovery can inspire both other service users and professionals alike*'.

I found this distinction helpful, but as I read the book I found it harder and harder to apply. Thus, I could easily see Florence Nightingale as the founder of scientific nursing and Rachel Perkins as having made a monumental contribution to thinking and practice in mental health services in England in the last 40 years. Similarly, I could see that without Charles Darwin, complete with his anxiety and depression, we might have had a very different view of our position in the animal kingdom and without Winston Churchill, with his own very peculiar mix of psychopathology, the history of the 20th century would have been very different.

However, I also felt that I could not overlook the personal struggle of everyone in the book to find meaning and purpose and to provide inspiration. I also felt uncomfortable about making judgements as to what was most likely to be of '*greater good for all humanity*'. Who knows what the impact of Michelle McNary's new film will be, or Bose Dania's next book of poetry? My conclusion was that all these individuals are 'heroes' in both the Greek and the 'routine' sense and that Patricia Deegan was right in trying to get all her students to '*try and see each individual as a hero*'.

What everyone in this book has in common is their direct experience of mental health problems and the effects, albeit some positive and some not so, of these experiences on their lives. But what the stories show is how different these experiences are for each person. In the best services we have always tried to take account of the huge differences between people, not just in terms of the nature of their problems, but also in their thinking, their internal worlds and their beliefs about what might be helpful for them and what might not. This book sets these out in their bewildering variety. It feels like an impossible challenge to adequately acknowledge this diversity and, of course, it is. But only by accepting it and recognising our limitations can professionals actually begin to face up to each encounter as a new beginning. Once we start to rely on familiar stereotypes and categories then we are lost. Thus, we need to continually celebrate the variety and ingenuity of people's own attempts to manage their conditions, from Abraham Lincoln's formulation of the three major factors that affect those of a nervous disposition: '*stressful events, isolation, idleness and bad weather*' (see Chapter 4) to Augusto Mello's wonderful and mysterious, '*power of the slow*' (see Chapter 19). These are certainly not 'tools' or 'models' of general application, they are hard-bitten nuggets of understanding chiselled out of the experience of life. Such is the wonderful flexibility of the human condition.

It is also clear that the people in the book have many different explanations for why they have experienced mental health problems and what might be helpful in dealing with them. Rufus May is clearly opposed to labelling his experiences as, '*a biological problem called schizophrenia, which needed to be suppressed with heavy doses of stupefying psychiatric drugs*'. On the other hand, for Peter Chadwick, '*a tiny amount of haloperidol ... seemed to take away barriers to the emergence of real-self rather than turning me into someone I'm not*'.

Q. Who is correct? A. Both are (of course). As Glenn Roberts points out (see Chapter 20) medication may have a contribution to make to supporting recovery, but the response is always individual and for each individual it must be seen within the overall context of their life. This is why it is important for service users and psychiatrists to work on their communication skills to achieve more genuinely '*shared*' decision-making regarding medication regimes (Deegan & Drake, 2006).

Families (and professionals) also appear repeatedly in both positive and negative roles. Many of the contributors describe harrowing stories of ill-treatment, childhood abuse or simple, long-term neglect from family members which they attribute as the cause of many of their problems. Many can also identify encounters with mental health professionals, including psychiatrists, which have been unhelpful and, at times frankly damaging. On the other hand, for every person who can tell a story of abuse at the hands of their family, there is also someone (sometimes the same person) who believes firmly that the positive aspects of their current recovery would not be possible without the support of family members. Similarly, several people identify particular professionals (also including psychiatrists) without whose help their recovery journeys would not have been possible. What these key figures all seem to have contributed most importantly is hope. Time and again different authors speak of the fundamental value of having people that believe in you and your potential at times when you find it difficult to believe in yourself. Sometimes this is family members, sometimes it is professionals, and often it is 'peers'. Of course, this is obvious. We all know that sometimes we need to rely on others to get us through hard times. It is natural and human. It is therefore a great pity if this is something that many professionals apparently find so difficult to do.

What other contributions might professionals make to supporting recovery? Most of the mental health professionals in this book – Peter Chadwick, Emma Harding, Rachel Perkins, Rufus May and Glenn Roberts – seem to be fairly sceptical of much that passes for mental health professional expertise. They stress the importance of professionals being prepared to use their own life experiences, in addition to their professional training. The concept of the 'wounded healer' is natural to all those who accept their 'wounds' as an ordinary part of life's experiences, but it is more unusual among most professionals. They also argue that we seem to have lost the balance between technical competence and human qualities. This means a different approach to the use of 'evidence-based' approaches; different kinds of training and management of staff; and different kinds of selection and management processes. It may even mean going beyond traditional thinking about the balance between mental health professionals and staff who are 'experientially qualified' (ie. people who are trained and employed to use their lived experience to help others with mental health problems) in the workforce. These challenges are set out in our most recent analysis of the organisational barriers to supporting recovery (Shepherd *et al*, 2010).

One of the other common themes in these narratives is the importance of the search for personal meaning. Our scientific explanations of complex mental health problems are fragmentary and poorly integrated and based almost entirely on results from group studies. They will therefore always need to be interpreted for individuals and this always means a degree of probabilistic inference. So, people *can* legitimately hold very different views regarding causation of mental illness and people *can* disagree: this is not a problem. What is a problem is if professionals begin to dispute the idea that everyone needs to have a set of explanations that make personal sense, rather than conforms to scientific understanding. This is particularly true of symptoms. For example, Peter Chadwick is convinced that, '*psychotic episodes and psychotic symptoms ....* [are not] .... *empty speech acts*'. Similarly, Emma Harding believes, '*that however nonsensical someone's beliefs sound, if you listen enough they actually do make sense*'. These professionals are engaged in the same quest described by non-professionals like Stuart Baker-Brown who is, '*constantly in search for the possible truth behind my own symptoms*'. The role of professionals in this quest is to support it and to offer their views, based on their training and their life experience, in the hope that this might be helpful. It is not to dictate answers.

When supported in this way – by family, friends, professionals, whoever – what people then choose to do with their lives, their 'pathways' to recovery, are unique and often extraordinary. For me, there was a strong theme of what might be called 'creativity' in these pathways, both in the artistic sense, but also in a broader, intellectual sense. Thus, several of the contributors described the importance of writing, performing, film-making and poetry in supporting their recovery. The professionals represented here have all made highly creative contributions to our understanding of the lives of people with mental health problems and how services might better respond to them. In addition, nearly all the contributors showed a common desire to share their experiences as an example to others. This is not 'boasting'; it is simply trying to demonstrate to others that they are capable of more in their lives than they might think. This is 'inspiration'.

Why is 'inspiration' so important in this context? Surely, everyone agrees that there is a certain heroism in the lives of people who are struggling with mental health problems? Well, everyone does not. There is still a unique stigma attached to mental health problems and, in the general public 'heroism' is not an adjective most people would attach to living with severe mental illness. For most people, 'heroes' are soldiers struggling to live with the trauma of injury sustained in war or conflict; or people with chronic physical disease, or brain tumours. For the general public, 'mental illness' continues to attract almost entirely negative reactions and expectations. This experience of stigma is written deeply in the lives of everyone in this book. For them, it is not an abstract, sociological concept; it is part of their everyday reality. They experience ignorance and fear and the lowered expectations of teachers, employers, family and friends. Most disturbingly, they may encounter these same attitudes from the mental health professionals who are meant to be helping them. This is illustrated in a recent, brave paper by Graham Thornicroft and Diana Rose which addresses the discriminatory attitudes of some psychiatrists (2010) and is echoed in a study of the low expectations held by mental health professionals regarding the employment prospects of people with severe mental illness (Marwaha *et al*, 2008). In this climate it is not surprising that many people with mental health problems begin to believe these negative attitudes about themselves. Self-stigmatisation is common and it takes a huge leap of self-confidence not to accept what appears to be a general consensus. As Emma Harding puts it, '*Eventually* (hopefully) *madness will be accepted, expected and respected and people living with it won't stigmatise themselves, assume they are separate from 'normal' people or that they are alone*' (See Chapter 8). Hopefully Emma is right, but we are not there yet. This book points the way.

A final thought: recently we have been reminded of the darker side of social encounters which place care staff in an unregulated position of power and authority over others. The result is abuse and this has always been the case. Apart from more effective, local monitoring and supervision of these situations, this could not happen if staff retained the feeling of excitement and discovery that usually characterises our first meetings with people we have been asked to see. As Jerome Carson comments when Gordon McManus was referred to his team, '*Fortunately for me, I was the one asked to see him*'. I found this simple assertion of values both moving and challenging. This book opens our eyes again to the rich voyages of discovery that we are sometimes privileged to share with the extraordinary people described in its pages. I thank the authors for bringing them together and I thank the contributors for sharing their lives.

References

Deegan PE & Drake RE (2006) Shared decision making and medication management in the recovery process. *Psychiatric Services* **57** 1636–1639.

Marwaha S, Balachandra S & Johnson S (2009) Clinicians' attitudes to the employment of people with psychosis. *Social Psychiatry Psychiatric Epidemiology* **44** (5) 349–360.

Shepherd G, Boardman J & Burns M (2010) Implementing recovery: a methodology for organisational change. London, Centre for Mental Health. Available at: www.centreformentalhealth.org.uk (accessed July 2011).

Thornicroft G, Rose D & Mehta N (2010) Discrimination against people with mental illness: what can psychiatrists do? *Advances in Psychiatric Treatment* **16** 53–59.

Bibliography

Repper J & Perkins R (2003) *Social Inclusion and Recovery*. London: Balliere Tindall.

Introduction

Jerome Carson, Elizabeth Wakely, Sophie Davies and Sarah Morgan

What is recovery?

'Recovery is an idea whose time has come.' (Shepherd *et al*, 2008)

The influential Sainsbury's Centre for Mental Health report *Making Recovery a Reality* provides the above quotation. Yet papers on recovery have been appearing in the literature since Patricia Deegan's first paper on the topic (Deegan, 1988). The most widely accepted definition of recovery was provided by the American clinical psychologist, Professor Bill Anthony. He defined recovery as:

'Recovery is described as a deeply personal, unique process of changing one's attitudes, values, feelings, goals, skills and/or roles. It is a way of living a satisfying, hopeful and contributing life even with the limitations caused by illness. Recovery involves the development of new meaning and purpose in life as one grows beyond the catastrophic effects of mental illness.' (Anthony, 1993)

A much more succinct definition is provided by Gordon McManus, one of the contributors to this volume. Gordon defines recovery as *'coping with your illness and having a meaningful life'* (McManus *et al*, 2009).

Unusually for the mental health field, the term recovery has been embraced by many service users, mental health professional groups, mental health lobby groups and even governments across the world. Recovery is now an established element of government policy (NIMHE, 2005; Department of Health, 2009). This is not to say that the issues raised by the adoption of the recovery approach have been received uncritically. Two workshops on the theme of recovery, hosted by the Social Perspectives Network and Mind, showed significant disagreements among stakeholders (Social Perspectives Network, 2007; Mind, 2008). For instance, one participant criticised the *'narrow focus on employment as the Holy Grail of Recovery,'* (Mind, 2008).

Considerable scepticism about the benefits and wisdom of the recovery approach can also be found among frontline workers. Typical comments include the following: '*We shouldn't be delivering medication to patients if we are operating a recovery model. They should be coming here to the team base to collect their medication!*'

The reception of recovery from service users has not always been positive either. One commented about one of us, saying that Jerome '*had got hooked into the recovery model, which seems to be based on a talk given by Dr Patricia Deegan some time ago. From a brief look at her on the web, she seems to have created an industry around her ideas. She also claims to have had psychotic illness when she was a teenager. P and I are rather mistrustful of all this especially when his psychologist says it is the big thing in mental health circles these days. Speaking for ourselves we've never seen anyone who has been to the places we have recover. The most people can do is more or less survive at home with the occasional spell as an inpatient.*'

Another commented, '*As you know I do not believe in, or accept the concept of the so-called recovery model and wish to have nothing at all to do with it!*' You cannot please all of the people all of the time. Many service users are also sceptical that the keenness with which many managers have rushed to embrace recovery means that they may be discharged from services, as they are presumed to have 'recovered.'

Clinical versus personal recovery

Historically mental health services have focused on clinical recovery as the main outcome of psychiatric services (Liberman & Kopelowicz, 2005). In the view of these authors, recovery is defined operationally as a two year period of symptom remission, engagement in work or education, independent living, good family relations, being involved in recreational activities and having a satisfying social network. By these criteria, very few people in our own local recovery and support service in southwest Lambeth could be said to have 'recovered'. Other authors stress the importance of personal recovery (Slade, 2009a; 2009b; Bird *et al*, 2011).

According to Mike Slade, personal recovery is based on two beliefs:

1. '*That recovery is something worked towards and experienced by the person with mental illness. It is not something that services can do to the person. The contribution of staff is to support the person in their journey toward recovery.*'

2. *'That the journey of recovery is individual. The best way of supporting an individual's journey will vary from person to person.'* (2009a)

Along with other colleagues, Mike Slade is conducting a very large study of how to implement personal recovery into community mental health teams. They describe the aim of their intervention as the following: *'The primary aim of the intervention is to support the personal recovery of people who use services. This will involve striving towards their goals, with partnership support where needed from staff. The type of support and the way it is provided by staff will be guided by the person's unique strengths, values and treatment preferences.'* (Bird *et al*, 2011)

What has driven the recovery movement?

Some authors have argued that the impetus towards recovery has come from the findings of long-term outcome studies of schizophrenia (see reviews by Dorrer, 2006; Warner, 2009). These studies conducted in several countries have shown after long-term follow-ups that the majority of people given a diagnosis of schizophrenia go on to make complete recovery from the condition. Other authors have argued that the drive towards recovery has come from the service user movement, which they say is, *'a grassroots movement of the disenfranchised that has placed itself apart from the human services professions,'* (Resnick & Rosenheck, 2006). There is no doubt that the service user literature has been central to our understanding of what recovery means for individuals (Deegan, 1996; Leibrich, 1999; Chandler & Hayward, 2009; Davidson and Lynn, 2009; Cordle *et al*, 2011). Indeed some researchers have used the service user literature to shape their understanding of recovery (Andresen *et al*, 2003; 2006). From their analysis of service user accounts, Retta Andresen and her colleagues have suggested there are four key processes in recovery. First is the restoration of hope; second is the development of a positive sense of identity; third is bringing meaning into people's lives; fourth is encouraging a sense of personal agency, responsibility and self-determination. This book falls within this developing service user literature on recovery.

Aims of this book

There are two main aims of this book. The first is to show how five major historical figures could be considered to be mental health recovery heroes and how their lives were in fact enhanced by their mental illnesses. The second is to provide narratives from contemporary mental health recovery heroes, which might inspire professionals working with people with long-term mental health problems, their carers, and most importantly service users themselves. Both the historical and contemporary individuals presented here are considered to be mental health recovery heroes.

Recovery heroes: where the idea came from?

There were three main sources that inspired looking at the concept of mental health recovery heroes and writing this book.

1. The heroic literature in storytelling

The term 'hero' derives from the Greek 'heros'. It was a term first used in Greek mythology and folklore. Heroes, or indeed heroines, were individuals who in the face of danger or adversity showed either courage or self-sacrifice for some greater good of all humanity. Heroes and heroic tales can be seen across all historical periods and cultures. The American psychiatrist, Scott-Peck, talks of the routine heroism of human beings (1991). Heroism can be found everywhere. Lorna Catford and Michael Ray, in their book *The Path of the Everyday Hero*, compare each of our life journeys with that of a hero's journey. They argue that each of us is confronted by five major challenges in our lives which are as follows. First, discovering and pursuing our true purpose in life; second, bringing love into our lives; third, living stress free in the here and now; fourth, achieving personal and professional balance; fifth, finding our way to prosperity (Catford & Ray, 1991). The authors' original definition of the term mental health recovery hero was, '*individuals whose journey of recovery can inspire both other service users and professionals alike,*' (Sen *et al*, 2009).

2. Seeing the individual service user as a hero

In her influential paper, *Recovery as a Journey of the Heart*, Patricia Deegan states that one of the ways she tries to help students working with service users is to get them to '*try and see the individual as a hero,*' (1996). She asks how each of us would be able to survive on a meagre income derived from benefits and cope with a major disability at the same time? She urges students to try and see service users as heroes who have survived.

3. Premila Trivedi's four recovery heroes

The mental health activist Premila Trivedi who worked in mental health services co-facilitated a one-day introductory workshop on recovery for staff from the London Boroughs of Lambeth and Southwark. She talked about her own four recovery heroes, which were Patricia Deegan, as aforementioned, and Mary Ellen Copeland, who is most associated with Wellness Recovery Action Planning (WRAP) and both of these women were from America. Her two British recovery heroes were Rachel Perkins and Peter Chadwick, both of whom feature in this volume.

It was a combination of the above factors that persuaded Jerome to approach Adam Pozner, the editor of *A Life in the Day* (now renamed as *Mental Health and Social Inclusion*). Jerome suggested to Adam that he consider commissioning a special issue of the journal on the concept of mental health recovery heroes. Adam felt it would be better to have a short series of papers in consecutive issues of the journal, and the first three papers that were produced were on Dolly Sen, Peter Chadwick and Gordon McManus. All three were asked to provide short biographies and were then interviewed by Sarah. Jerome then wrote a personal appraisal on each one. The last two papers in this series on Matthew Ward and Margaret Muir were written by Hannah Cordle and Jerome, and Jane Fradgley provided the art photography for each feature. Four of the five mental health recovery heroes were drawn from the local mental health service in southwest Lambeth where Jerome worked. Jerome went on to make the point that mental health recovery heroes could be found in all mental health services. Margaret Muir expanded this notion to say that anyone who had experienced major mental health problems was a hero, given what they had to do to survive. In this book, the accounts of the original five mental health recovery heroes have been amended and expanded upon and a further 10 accounts taken from across Britain have been added. Some of these individuals will be already well known to readers, others will no doubt become better known as their own work expands.

Historical recovery heroes

The idea to look at historical mental health recovery heroes came about by chance. Jerome ran a recovery group at his local community mental health team (Morgan & Carson, 2009) and Liz had started attending this group. Having seen a number of presentations by group members, Jerome asked Liz if she would be willing to give one herself. Liz had worked for many years as a history teacher.

How could we combine history and mental health? The answer was provided by reading a paper by Campbell & Jones (2009), which was produced as part of the national Time to Change campaign. In this short paper, the authors asked us to imagine what our world would have been like if their 'fantastic five' had been barred from taking their rightful place in society by discrimination against people with mental health problems? Their fantastic five were Winston Churchill, Florence Nightingale, Charles Darwin, Marie Curie and Abraham Lincoln. I asked Liz if she would be prepared to give a presentation on these individuals to the recovery group. Liz not only presented the stories of Winston Churchill, Florence Nightingale and Charles Darwin, but she advanced a different thesis. She argued that these three individuals' lives were in fact enhanced by their respective mental health problems. Some months after this, I again approached Adam Pozner and asked if he would like us to provide him with some historical recovery heroes to follow on from our previous series of contemporary recovery heroes. He again agreed and we provided him with accounts on Churchill, Nightingale and Darwin. We asked him if we could do a fourth and final account on Isaac Newton, who was not one of the five in Campbell and Jones' original series, but was someone whose life intrigued both Liz and myself. Again we have extended these accounts in the chapters in this book and we have also added an account of Abraham Lincoln who was not featured in our series of four papers.

The work on historical recovery heroes has been one of the most interesting pieces of work that Jerome has engaged in. It brings to bear the expertise of an historian, Liz, with that of a mental health professional, Jerome, in a unique collaboration. In this task we have been ably assisted by Paul Harrington, the librarian at Lambeth Hospital, who has conducted literature searches for us on these famous people. Sheila Watson has obtained key journal papers for us. In preparing our paper on Florence Nightingale we were also grateful for discussions we had on the nature of her illness with Dr Robin Stott, Helen Wakely and also Kirsteen Nixon from the Florence Nightingale Museum.

The significance of the historical and contemporary mental health recovery heroes

There is no doubting the key contributions made to our society by people like Isaac Newton, Charles Darwin, Florence Nightingale, Winston Churchill and Abraham Lincoln. What is less well known in almost all their cases is the degree to which their lives were shaped by their mental health problems. Even well read colleagues expressed surprise when Jerome mentioned Liz and he were looking at the mental health problems of figures like Newton and Darwin. Churchill's problems with depression, his so-called Black Dog, have been well documented (Storr, 1989). Florence Nightingale is best known for her work in the Crimean War and her contributions to the development of nursing, but most people are totally oblivious to the fact that she was housebound for three decades after she returned from the Crimea (Bostridge, 2008). Only one of our five historical mental health recovery heroes, Abraham Lincoln, has had books written specifically on his mental health problems (Burlingame, 1997; Shenk, 2006). We have had to rely on journal papers and parts of biographies to discover more about the mental health problems of these famous individuals. It is too early to discern if our accounts of these famous people have either caused others to re-appraise their views of the role of mental health problems in their lives, or whether bringing their problems into the public domain has inspired people who suffer with mental health problems. There are different aspects of each of the five's individual stories that can inspire others. To mention but one example, Charles Darwin did not do a day's paid work in his life. He survived entirely on an annual income provided to him by his father (Desmond & Moore, 2009). The fact that each of these eminent individuals suffered with long-term mental health problems will hopefully offer encouragement to readers currently experiencing mental health problems.

To turn to our contemporary mental health recovery heroes, we have featured 15 accounts of individuals from a diverse set of backgrounds. Some of these individuals work as mental health professionals themselves, Rachel Perkins, Rufus May, Glenn Roberts and Emma Harding. Others are heavily involved in educating service users and mental health professionals about recovery, Peter Bullimore, Dolly Sen, Andrew Voyce and Augusto D Mello. Peter Chadwick used to be an academic and continues to write about mental health and recovery using his own experience of psychosis as a way of connecting academic psychology with our understanding of psychotic processes (Chadwick, 2011a; 2011b). Matthew Ward is an actor who has also been involved in using his acting talents to try and educate people about recovery (Ward *et al*, 2010). Michelle McNary is a film maker who has just produced an inspiring film featuring the recovery journeys of four individuals from south London, all of whom have been given a diagnosis of psychosis. Michelle has presented these four individuals as recovery philosophers (see www.slam.nhs.uk/patients/recovery.aspx). Bose Dania, now a mother, has moved from professional dancing to writing poetry as part of her recovery journey. Gordon McManus has gone from being a communist revolutionary to a mental health revolutionary with his writings on recovery. Margaret Muir has developed an interest in photography as a way of finding a new perspective in her retirement years. Finally, Stuart Baker-Brown became a Churchill Fellow and travelled to Everest Base camp bringing back some wonderful photography, and continuing to share this journey with others though his presentations for over a decade since his first visit.

Each of the 15 contemporary recovery heroes has lived experience of mental health problems. Each has contributed to our developing understanding of recovery. Each has made a unique contribution to the field and it is our genuine hope that reading these brief accounts of their stories will inspire our readers.

References

Andresen R, Oades L & Caputi P (2003) The experience of recovery from schizophrenia: towards an empirically validated stage model. *Australian and New Zealand Journal of Psychiatry* **37** (5) 586–594.

Andresen R Caputi P & Oades L (2006) Stages of Recovery Instrument: development of a measure of recovery from severe mental illness. *Australian and New Zealand Journal of Psychiatry* **40** (10) 972–980.

Anthony W (1993) Recovery from mental illness: guiding vision of mental health service systems in 1990s. *Psychosocial Rehabilitation Journal* **16** (4) 11–23.

Bird V, Leamy M, Le Boutillier C, Williams J & Slade M (2011) *Refocus: Promoting recovery in community mental health services. Rethink Recovery Series: Volume 4.* London: Rethink.

Bostridge M (2008) *Florence Nightingale*. London: Penguin.

Burlingame M (1997) *The Inner World of Abraham Lincoln*. Chicago: University of Illinois Press.

Campbell A & Jones N (2009) *A World Without: The fantastic five*. London: Time to Change.

Catford L & Ray M (1991) *The Path of the Everyday Hero*. New York: Putnam.

Chadwick P (2011a) *From teddy boy to teddy bear, from barbells to bar-belle: on growth via psychosis, sin and love*. In: G McManus & J Carson (Eds) *From Communism to Schizophrenia and Beyond: One man's long march to recovery.* London: Whiting and Birch.

Chadwick P (2011b) *Does a psychotic episode ever do anybody any good*? In: G McManus & Carson J (Eds) *From Communism to Schizophrenia and Beyond: One man's long march to recovery*. London: Whiting and Birch.

Chandler R & Hayward M (Eds) (2009) *Voicing Psychotic Experiences: A reconsideration of recovery and diversity*. Brighton: Pavilion.

Cordle H, Fradgley J, Carson J, Holloway F & Richards P (2011) *Psychosis: Stories of recovery and hope*. London: Quay Books.

Davidson L & Lynn L (2009) (Eds) *Beyond the Storms: Reflections on personal recovery in Devon*. Exeter: Devon Partnership NHS Trust.

Deegan P (1988) Recovery: the lived experience of rehabilitation. *Psychosocial Rehabilitation Journal* **11** (4) 11–19.

Deegan P (1996) Recovery as a journey of the heart. *Psychiatric Rehabilitation Journal* **19** (3) 91–97.

Department of Health (2009) *New Horizons: Towards a shared vision for mental health*. London: Department of Health.

Desmond A & Moore J (2009) *Darwin*. London: Penguin.

Dorrer N (2006) *Evidence of Recovery: The ups and downs of longitudinal outcome research*. Glasgow: Scottish Recovery Network.

Leibrich J (1999) *A Gift of Stories*. Dunedin: University of Otago Press.

Liberman R & Kopelowicz A (2005) Recovery from schizophrenia: a concept in search of research. *Psychiatric Services* **56** (6) 735–742.

McManus G, Morgan S, Fradgley J & Carson J (2009) Recovery heroes – a profile of Gordon McManus. *A Life in the Day* **13** (4) 16–19.

Mind (2008) Life and times of a supermodel: the recovery paradigm for mental health. *MindThink Report 3*. London: Mind.

Morgan S & Carson J (2009) The recovery group: a service user and professional perspective. *Groupwork* **19** (1) 26–39.

National Institute for Mental Health in England (2005) *NIMHE Guiding Statement on Recovery*. London: Department of Health.

Resnick S & Rosenheck R (2006) Recovery and positive psychology: parallel themes and potential synergies. *Psychiatric Services* **57** (1) 120–123.

Scott-Peck M (1991) In: L Catford & M Ray (1991) *The Path of the Everyday Hero.* New York: Putnam.

Sen D, Morgan S & Carson J (2009) Recovery heroes – a profile of Dolly Sen. *A Life in the Day* **13** (2) 6–9.

Shenk J (2006) *Lincoln's Melancholy: How depression challenged a president and fuelled his greatness*. New York: Houghton Mifflin.

Shepherd G, Boardman J & Slade M (2008) *Making Recovery a Reality*. London: Sainsbury Centre for Mental Health.

Slade M (2009a) *100 Ways to Support Recovery: A guide for mental health professionals. Rethink Recovery Series: Volume 1*. London: Rethink.

Slade M (2009b) *Personal Recovery and Mental Illness; A guide for mental health professionals*. Cambridge: Cambridge University Press.

Social Perspectives Network (2007) *Whose Recovery is it Anyway?* London: Social Perspectives Network.

Storr A (1989) *Churchill's Black Dog and Other Phenomena of the Human Mind*. London: Harper Collins.

Ward M, Chander A, Robinson S, Farquharson Y & Carson J (2010) It's a one man show. *Mental Health Today* 32–33.

Warner R (2009) Recovery from schizophrenia and the medical model. *Current Opinion in Psychiatry* **22** (4) 374–380.

Part 1: Historical Recovery Heroes

Chapter 1

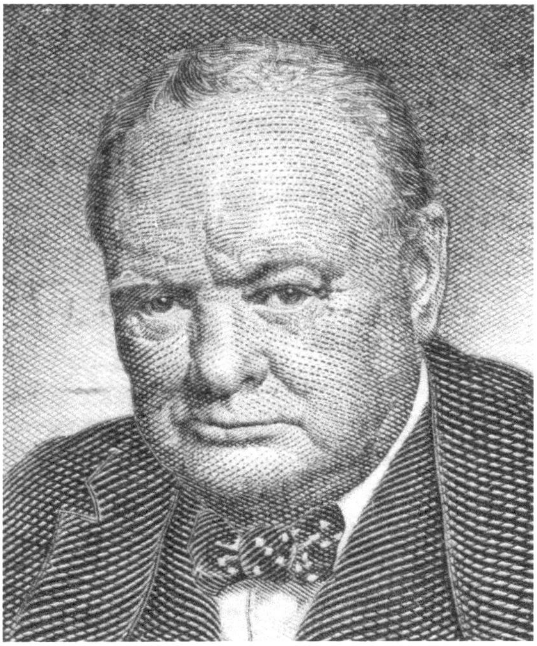

Winston Churchill

Summary

Winston Churchill is said by many to have been the greatest Englishman who ever lived, largely due to his leadership during the Second World War. Since his death in 1965, much more has become known about his lifelong battle with depression, his 'Black Dog', although it now seems more likely that he had bipolar disorder. In this chapter we argue that Churchill's mental illness may in fact have led to him being a better leader. Championed in 2006 in a statue dedicated by Rethink and most recently by the Time to Change campaign, Winston Churchill is a true recovery hero.

Upbringing and early life

Winston Leonard Spencer Churchill was born in 1874 to Lord Randolph Churchill, the third son of the seventh Duke of Marlborough, and Jennie (nee Jerome), the daughter of an American millionaire. He had one sibling, Jack, who was born five years later so effectively he was an only child during his formative years. His parents were very distant, with his father being a busy politician and his mother a young socialite. So the only person who saved him from emotional starvation was his nanny, Mary Anne Everest or 'Old Woom' as he called her. Indeed when she was dying in 1895, he returned from an army assignment in Cuba to stay with her for the last week of her life. He said of her, '*She had been my dearest and most intimate friend during the 20 years I had lived,*' (Churchill, 1930). He kept her photograph in his room until he died. By contrast, according to Randolph Churchill (1966), '*The neglect and lack of interest shown in him by his parents were remarkable, even judged by the standards of late Victorian and Edwardian days,*'.

Churchill was educated, as befitted one of his class, at prep schools and then at Harrow. He disliked school and felt very alone as can be seen from his letters to his mother in which he begged her to come and see him or to let him come home, to neither of which she acceded. He pleaded: '*Uncertainty is at all times perplexing. Write to me by return of post please!!! I love you so much dear Mummy and know you love me too much to disappoint me. Do write to me to tell me what you intend to do. I must come home, I feel I must,*' (June, 1887, cited in Churchill, 1930). Physically, he was small and slight, but he was determined to prove himself and he excelled at fencing. He said this about his school years, '*...these years form not only the least agreeable, but the only barren and unhappy period of my life ... All my contemporaries and even younger boys seemed far better at the games and at the lessons. It is not pleasant to feel oneself so completely outclassed and left behind at the beginning of the race,*' (Churchill, 1930). Academically he was not a success although he was good at history and English, both of which were to stand him in good stead later in life. He left school in 1893 to go to Sandhurst from where he joined the 4th Queen's Own Hussars.

Career and achievements

Churchill pursued a military career from 1895 to 1900, although he had a brief break when he became a war correspondent for the *Morning Post* in the Boer War. Some of this time he spent as a prisoner of war in Pretoria, from which he escaped but the experience gave him an understanding of the suffering of prisoners. In 1900, he entered politics where he had a varying degree of success, switching between Liberal and Conservative parties and holding various Cabinet posts between 1908 and 1929. This included being Chancellor of the Exchequer (1924–9), during which time he supervised sterling's return to the Gold Standard (1925) and made himself very unpopular in some quarters by his belligerent and uncompromising stance towards the miners and in the General Strike of 1926. But after the Conservative defeat at the General Election of 1929, he was out of office and the 1930s have been described by historians as his 'wilderness years,' (Gilbert, 1981). He thought his political career was at an end and this led to a period of depression and despair, during which he found solace in his painting and he became an accomplished artist. However with the outbreak of World War II in September 1939, he entered the War Cabinet as First Lord of the Admiralty – a position which he had held earlier but resigned from in 1915 after the disaster of the Dardanelles expedition. Then in May 1940, aged 65, at a time when most people would be contemplating retirement, he became Prime Minister. This was on the resignation of Neville Chamberlain who had been the architect of the policy of appeasement (i.e. giving in to Hitler's demands), a policy with which Churchill had profoundly disagreed throughout the 1930s when he constantly demanded rearmament as Hitler's ambitions for European domination became clear. When Churchill became Prime Minister, as he had foreseen, most of Europe was under Nazi control. Norway had just been overrun and in June 1940 France would fall, leaving Britain alone to face the Nazi threat and very likely invasion by German troops from across the Channel, particularly after the ignominious, if heroic, evacuation of British troops from Dunkirk in the same month. However against what seemed like overwhelming odds Churchill was determined not just to resist but to win and in the end he did exactly that. His attitude can be seen in a few excerpts from his speeches in the House of Commons.

'*I have nothing to offer but blood, toil, tears and sweat ... victory at all costs.*' (Hansard, May 13, 1940)

'*We shall go on to the end ... we shall fight on the beaches ... we shall never surrender.*' (Hansard, June 4, 1940a)

'*Hitler knows that he will have to break us in these islands or lose the war. If we can stand up to him, all Europe may be free and the life of the world may move forward into broad sunlit uplands.*' (Hansard, June 8, 1940b)

Churchill's speeches and broadcasts continued throughout the war. These displayed his ruthless determination, his stubborn refusal to admit defeat and his message of defiance and hope to encourage the country to endure the hardships and fight to win. As CP Snow commented, *'That voice was our hope. It was the voice of will and strength incarnate,'* (Snow, 1969). Throughout the war, Churchill was the man who oversaw all the military effort, such as the defeat of the Germans in North Africa in 1942 through the D Day landings in June 1944, to the final defeat of Germany. Much of this was certainly controversial, then as now, as he fell out with and overruled many of his commanders in the field and his advisors; and the bombing of Dresden in February 1945 is seen by many as an unworthy and unnecessary act of retaliation and revenge. But Britain, under his leadership, won the war. At the same time Churchill also oversaw all that was going on at home, inspiring the people to take whatever the Germans threw at them, to suffer rationing and shortages and come through with the 'bulldog spirit'. So, after terrible air raids during the Blitz in the winter of 1940–41, he would be there the next day inspecting the damage and rallying the people as well as broadcasting messages of hope and encouragement and working in his underground headquarters. He seemed to do this with boundless and frenetic energy working for more than 18 hours a day, either from his office or from home, maddening his staff and his family with his impatience and demands. A civil servant described his attitude thus, *'The Prime Minister has determined that we shall die in the last ditch, and there is no one inclined to say him nay,'* (Snow, 1969). And as Snow himself says *'Churchill ... was an aristocrat, but he would have beggared his class and his friends, and everyone else too, if that were the price of the country coming through,'* (1969). His achievement was, to quote Campbell & Jones, that his *'leadership ensured the survival of freedom and democracy – it is as awesomely simple as that,'* (2009).

After the war, his career took a downturn. Labour won the General Election of 1945 and, although Churchill became Prime Minister again between 1950 and 1953, things were never the same for him. He died aged 90 in January 1965 and was given a 'lying in state' in Westminster Hall and a state funeral in St. Paul's Cathedral. According to his personal physician, Lord Moran, the last five years of his life had been spent in deep depression.

Mental illness aspects

'I have achieved a great deal to achieve nothing in the end.' (Churchill, 1967)

This remark, made by Churchill to his daughter on one birthday towards the end of his life, is characteristic of depressive thinking. It is well known that Churchill suffered with depression, which he referred to as his Black Dog, as it is well-documented by him and by those around him. These often intense and prolonged depressive episodes began in his youth and were closely linked to what was going on in his life, for instance his loneliness at school, his loss of office and prestige after the Dardanelles fiasco – when he first took up painting – and in his 'wilderness years' of the 1930s. As well as having a genetic factor, '*... the cyclothymic temperament ... was part of the Churchill inheritance,*' (Storr, 1989), his depression can be traced back to his experiences of emotional deprivation in his childhood and adolescence, during which he also developed compensatory traits such as his vaunting and compulsive ambition and his determination to show moral and physical courage. He also had problems dealing with hostility. '*Winston Churchill's obstinacy, resentment of authority, and wilfulness were manifest very early in his life,*' (Storr, 1989). This difficulty in dealing with hostility leads some depressives to seek out opponents in the external world and for Churchill this found perfect release and resolution when he was confronted by Hitler, whom he regarded as evil incarnate and upon whom he could unleash all his enormous aggressiveness.

The more contemporary view is that Churchill was not just depressed, but that he had bipolar disorder. His close friend Lord Beaverbrook said, '*he was always at the top of the wheel of confidence or at the bottom of an intense depression*'. And, to Lady Violet Bonham Carter, Churchill himself said, '*We are all worms. But I do believe that I am a glow-worm,*' (Bonham Carter, 1967), which as Storr comments shows '*self-abasement and self-glorification in a single phrase,*' (1989). There were many manic features in his behaviour. As well as his enormous vitality, he showed a lack of inhibition, for instance receiving civil servants when naked in his bathtub, and he had a disdainful attitude towards other people and their opinions, not only in the House of Commons but also in his own personal relationships. He was noted for his extravagance, his belligerence and combativeness and his unwavering belief in his own invincibility and in his own destiny as a great man. '*This cannot be accident, it must be design. I was kept for this job.*' (Moran, 1966).This last statement encapsulates another aspect of the bipolar mind: the blurring of the line between fantasy and reality. As Lord Moran commented, '*... it was the inner world of make-believe in which Winston found reality,*' (Morgan, 1966) and at the age of 65, Churchill's fantasy became reality. He had a heroic mission to fulfil, he believed in himself entirely and, because of his complete conviction, he was able to convey his inspiration to others and override all opposition.

What Churchill would have made of this analysis of him, we can only speculate. He had this to say about psychiatrists in a letter to John Anderson, '*I am sure it would be sensible to restrict as much as possible the work of these gentlemen, who are capable of doing an immense amount of harm with what may very easily descend into charlatanry. The tightest hand should be kept over them, and they should not be allowed to quarter themselves among Fighting Services at the public expense.*' (Chickering & Förster)

Appraisal as a recovery hero

It seems hard to conceive that the greatest Englishman who ever lived suffered with long-term mental illness, yet there is no doubt Churchill did. Since his death, his status as a mental health recovery hero has grown. Churchill was one of the 'fantastic five' chosen by Alastair Campbell and Nigel Jones as part of the Time to Change anti-stigma campaign (2009). Drawing on work that showed 60% of employers would not employ someone with a history of mental illness, they argued that if the 'fantastic five' had been subject to discrimination, the world would be a very different place today. In 2006, Rethink commissioned a statue of Churchill in a straitjacket. In a press statement they commented: '*The message we want to portray is that it is possible to recover from mental illness and overcome it and be successful – because Churchill is an example of someone who was able to do that.*'

Storr comments that '*Perhaps the most remarkable feature of Churchill's psychology is that on the whole the defences he employed against depression proved so successful,*' (1989). These included writing, painting and, perhaps more unusually for someone of an aristocratic background, bricklaying, along with over indulgence in food, alcohol and cigars.

Conclusion

On the one hand it could be argued that in spite of his mental health problems, especially his debilitating depression which laid him low and rendered him inactive for long periods, Churchill achieved greatness in leading his country to victory in World War II. But, on the other hand, it could be more cogently argued that it was because of his mental health problems that Churchill achieved what he did. First, his experience of depression enabled him to comprehend and sympathise with the despair that the English people felt not only in 1940 but also throughout the years of wartime austerity and deprivation. This helped him to express their suffering, boost their morale and offer them hope and inspiration. Second, and perhaps more importantly, it was the manic aspects of his disorder that gave him the trump card. As Storr (1989) says so succinctly '*... had he been a stable and equable man, he could never have inspired the nation. In 1940, when all the odds were against Britain, a leader of sober judgement might well have concluded that we were finished*'. But not Churchill.

References

Bonham Carter V (1967) *Winston Churchill As I Knew Him*. London: Pan.

Campbell A & Jones N (2009) *A World Without the Fantastic Five*. London: Time to Change.

Chickering R & Förster S (2003) *The Shadows of Total War*. Cambridge: Cambridge University Press.

Churchill R (1966) *Winston S Churchill*. London: Heinemann.

Churchill S (1967) *A Thread in the Tapestry*. London: Andre Deutsch.

Churchill W (1930) *My Early Life a Roving Commission*. London: Thornton Butterworth.

Gilbert M (1981) *Churchill: The wilderness years*. London: MacMillan.

Hansard (May 1940) Vol 360, Cols 1501–1525.

Hansard (June 1940a) Vol 361, Cols 787–798.

Hansard (June 1940b) Vol 362, Cols 51–64.

Moran Lord (1966) *Churchill: The struggle for survival 1940–1965*. London: Constable.

Snow CP (1969) *Variety of Men*. Harmondsworth: Penguin.

Storr A (1989) *Churchill's Black Dog and Other Phenomena of the Human Mind*. London: Harper Collins.

Chapter 2

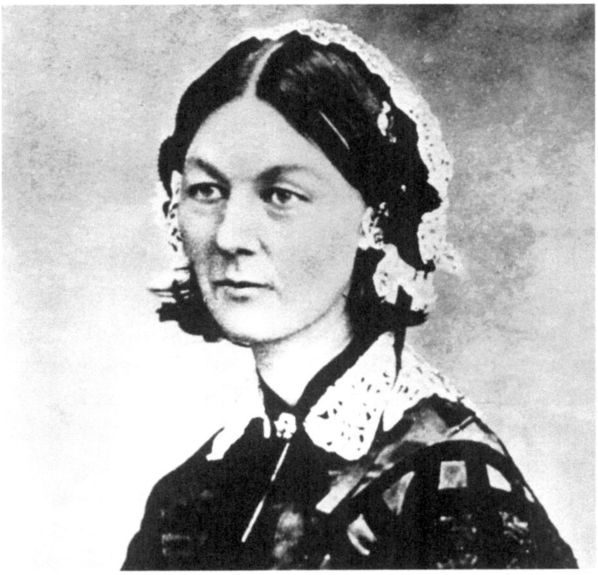

Florence Nightingale

Summary

Florence Nightingale was one of the most influential women of the 19th century. She is most closely associated with the Crimean War and the subsequent development of the nursing profession. Before she went to the Crimea, she had experienced episodes of depression. While in the Crimea she contracted brucellosis and, although she returned to England a national heroine, she lived the life of an invalid for several decades. Despite her physical and mental health problems, she produced over 200 reports, pamphlets and books, not just on nursing, but on a wide variety of other topics. This phenomenal productivity has led some authors to suggest she may have had bipolar disorder.

Upbringing and early life

Florence Nightingale was born in 1820 and was the second daughter of a wealthy landowner, William Nightingale and his wife Fanny. Her sister Parthenope, known as Parthe, was just a year older and with her she had a somewhat difficult relationship due, it would seem, not just to the usual sibling rivalry but also to Parthe's desire to dominate and control her more intelligent and somewhat wayward younger sister. During her childhood Florence was very close to her father who taught her, along with Parthe, Greek, Latin, French, German, Italian, history, philosophy and mathematics. In the last she showed considerable talent in collecting and analysing data, an ability which was to be very important in her later life. Her mother, while quite a dominant figure, preferred to concentrate on religion and on trying to find her a suitable husband. In the latter Fanny was disappointed as Florence turned down at least three proposals of marriage, the most promising being from Richard Monckton Milnes (later 1st Baron Houghton); but Florence considered a woman's life wasted in marriage and motherhood. Most of her childhood was spent at the family's country houses, where she first discovered her talent in caring for the poor and the sick, as an antidote to the intense boredom and consequent depression she experienced in her conventional upbringing.

In February 1837, just before her 17th birthday, she had a call from God to some as yet unspecified task: '*God spoke to me and called me to His service,*' (Bostridge, 2008) and by 1844 she had decided that this service lay in nursing. However, this was vigorously opposed by her parents who considered it totally unsuitable for a lady. Florence recorded in a note, '*Forgive me, O God, and let me die, this day let me die,*' (Bostridge, 2008).

In the autumn of 1847 she suffered what would today be called a nervous breakdown. As a result, she was sent to Italy to recuperate and it was there in November to December 1847 that she met the politician Sidney Herbert, a meeting that was to change her life. In early March 1850, she experienced several more calls from God, writing in her diary entry of March 7 '*God called me in the morning and asked me "Would I do good for Him, for Him alone without the reputation?"*' and she was once more on the verge of breakdown because of the conflict between her duty to her family and serving God. However, in July 1850 she paid a two week visit to the Lutheran community at Kaiserwerth in Germany where she saw at first hand the work being done for the poor and the sick and the training that the nurses received, and this inspired her. It was because she then experienced a further depressive episode, recording in her diary for 30th December, '*I have no desire now but to die,*' that in 1851 her father agreed that she could go to Kaiserwerth to study from July to October. Then in August 1853, with her father's consent she took up the post of Superintendent of the Establishment for Gentlewomen during Illness in Upper Harley Street. She was now nursing.

Career and achievements

The Crimea: The Lady with the Lamp

Soon after the outbreak of the Crimean War in March 1854, reports of the terrible conditions and neglect that wounded soldiers were experiencing began to reach Britain. *The Times* correspondent, William Russell, asked '*Are there no devoted women among us, able and willing to go forth to minister to the sick and suffering soldiers of the East in the hospitals of Scutari?*' (1854). In October, thanks to her friendship with Sidney Herbert (by then Secretary for War), Florence and 38 nurses were sent out.

On her arrival Florence found that '*There are no vessels for water or utensils of any kind; no soap, towels or clothes ... the men lying in their uniforms, stiff and covered with filth ... their persons covered with vermin,*' (Bostridge, 2008) and that men were dying as much from disease as from their wounds, which she attributed to lack of organisation and training, a lack of supplies, poor diet and poor hygiene. So she set about remedying the situation. She ordered medicine and bandages, equipment, food, clothing, blankets, utensils, tools (even nails) and lamps; and she set up a laundry and a proper kitchen. The system of purveying, or army supply, was inefficient and she had to fight endless battles to get anything done, which made her many enemies. However, despite her best efforts the death toll in the Scutari hospitals rose during the winter of 1854–55 to unprecedented heights reaching 4007 in February 1855, which was over 50% of the patients admitted. This was, as revealed by a Sanitary Commission sent out from London in March 1855, caused because of bad sanitation, and when the drains and sewers were flushed out and ventilation improved, the mortality rate dropped dramatically to 2% by the end of the war in 1856. Florence herself refused to accept these findings, a refusal that was to cause her almost unbearable feelings of guilt later, and she continued to concentrate on organisation.

In spite of this preoccupation, with her tireless energy she still found time to look after her patients, which gave rise to intense gratitude among the soldiers: '*If there is any angels on Earth she is one … her delicate form gliding about amongst hundreds of great ruff soldiers … the looks of love and gratitude that they cast on her beloved face it always makes me good to see her …*' (Bostridge, 2008) and this led to her iconic status at home: '*When all the medical officers have retired for the night and sickness and darkness have settled down upon the miles of prostrate sick, she may be observed alone, with a little lamp in her hand, making her solitary rounds*' (Bostridge, 2008), hence the legend of the Lady with the Lamp. Then in 1855, Florence herself became desperately ill with 'Crimean Fever', subsequently diagnosed as brucellosis, and she returned home at the end of the war in 1856 an invalid.

After the Crimea

It was after her return to England that, arguably, Florence Nightingale's most important work was done despite recurrent bouts of illness, which kept her confined to her sickbed and made her increasingly reclusive. Her reclusiveness may also have been motivated partly by a desire, conscious or otherwise, to avoid her mother and sister who once more sought to gain some sort of control over her life. Fortunately her sister married in 1858 and had other preoccupations and it is probably significant that after mother died, in 1880, Florence became much more physically active and outgoing.

In the Crimea she had come to realise the many shortcomings in the army and civilian health systems and in 1857 she finally acknowledged the importance of sanitation and cleanliness and from then on this drove her to work on reform.

Florence is well known for reforming nursing: the publication of her *Notes on Nursing* in 1860 and the foundation of the Nightingale Training School for Nurses at St Thomas' Hospital in the same year led not only to the recognition of nursing as a respectable and valued profession but also to the establishment of nurses' training schools elsewhere, with Nightingale matrons and nurses going out to other hospitals.

However, her work went beyond this. Thanks to her ideas and her tireless campaigning, changes and innovations were made in both army and civilian hospitals, with improved medical training and good sanitation in barracks and hospitals. In her *Notes on Hospitals* (Nightingale, 1863) she advocated improved hospital design and building, making them light and airy with plenty of ventilation, which was incorporated into the building of the Royal Herbert Hospital for the Army at Woolwich and later in the new St Thomas' Hospital for civilians, opened in 1871. In 1867 the Metropolitan Poor Act was passed which reformed the organisation and made better provision for the nursing and care of the sick in workhouse infirmaries where previously conditions had been appalling. Mark Bostridge claims that this was '*the first explicit acknowledgement of the duty of the state to provide hospitals for the poor. Eighty years later the idea would come to fruition with the foundation of Britain's National Health Service,*' (Bostridge, 2008).

In other ways, too, Florence's ideas paved the way for the National Health Service as her interests extended to wider public health issues. These included midwifery (see her *Notes on Lying-in Institutions*, 1871) district nursing for local healthcare – in 1875 a District Nursing Association was formed in London (an idea which spread to other cities and in the 1890s) she encouraged the appointment of 'health commissioners' (the precursors of health visitors), to promote good health and prevent disease in the home, especially in rural districts. Her mission included not just the care and cure of the sick but also preventative medicine. In order to achieve these goals she put endless pressure on those in positions of power and influence and in her campaigning she produced numerous publications and reports, which made full use of her ability in collecting and analysing data to provide statistics, often presented as 'coxcombs' – an early form of the pie chart. Not content with concerns in Britain, she dedicated 40 years to the improvement of public health in India, concentrating at first on British soldiers and then expanding her commitment to the indigenous population, using all the same methods. In 1910, Florence Nightingale died a much venerated figure.

Feminism

Claims have been made that Florence Nightingale was also an early feminist, but this is to read history backwards. While certainly unconventional for her time, advancing nursing as a career for women and enjoying manipulating powerful men while remaining in the background, she never sought to enter the world of men. She did not believe that women should strive to become doctors, leaving such pioneering work to Elizabeth Garrett Anderson and Sophia Jex-Blake; and she had no time for the women's suffrage movement supporting neither Millicent Fawcett (sister of Elizabeth Garrett Anderson) and her peaceful suffragist movement nor the Pankhursts and their militant suffragettes. Her own views on this subject, apart from some correspondence with John Stuart Mill about removing restrictions on women having some sort of career, are to be found in a novel called Cassandra, unpublished in her lifetime and only seeing the light of day in 1928. It is in this novel that she rails against the tyranny of the Victorian family, a point of view entirely consistent with her stance throughout her lifetime.

Mental illness aspects

Unlike Churchill, who referred to his depression as his 'Black Dog', Florence Nightingale's mental health problems are much more contested. Campbell & Jones (2009) cite the work of the American psychiatrist Kathy Wisner who suggested that bipolar disorder was the cause of Nightingale's illness. Professor Wisner's diagnosis, '*Bipolar disorder, with psychotic features*' is presented in a case conference format, which details the historical evidence to back up this claim, (Wisner *et al*, 2005) but of course this is still to a large degree speculative rather than definitive.

In a conference paper given at one of her childhood homes, Embley, Hugh Small contrasts the range of theories that have been put forward to explain Florence Nightingale's illness post-Crimea (2010). Among the diagnoses that have been offered are neurasthenia, psychosomatic illness, feigned illness, physical invalidism due to brucellosis and he adds, most recently, bipolar disorder. Small, perhaps cynically, suggests that there is a theory that '*all heroes are bipolar*' (2010). To the above may be added chronic fatigue syndrome, more commonly referred to as ME (Jason *et al*, 2002) and post-traumatic stress disorder, '*complicated not just by survivor guilt but also by guilt over complicity in perpetuating the pestilence that carried off so many of her patients*' at Scutari (Mackowiack & Batten, 2008). Lytton Strachey's account additionally suggests that '*... in the real Miss Nightingale there was more that was interesting than in the legendary one; there was also less that was agreeable,*' (Strachey, 2009). This last point hints at personality issues, which certainly seem to have been apparent in her family relationships.

What is incontestable is Florence Nightingale's remarkable productivity after she returned from the Crimea despite her illnesses. Virginia Dunbar in a new foreword to *Notes on Nursing*, points out that '*her publications cover nursing, hospitals, administration, sanitation, health, statistics, philosophy, emigration, protection of aboriginal races, famine, punishment and discipline, conditions in India, thrift, birds and female suffrage,*' (Dunbar, 1969). She goes on to point out that Florence Nightingale's work was one of '*untiring thoroughness in reading, assembling, observing, testing and analysing of everything to be had on the subject at home or abroad and then lining up her facts with the obvious intent to produce action,'* (Dunbar, 1969). Bostridge drawing from one of Florence Nightingale's letters quotes, *'When I have work to do which must be finished by a certain time, I work sometimes 20 hours out of 24'*. He further points out that, '*... such a workload would have defeated most able bodied individuals, let alone someone suffering the effects of a chronic and debilitating illness,'* (Bostridge, 2008).

Appraisal as a recovery hero

Given that Florence Nightingale spent almost three decades after the Crimean War confined to her house and did not start walking again until she was in her 60s, her achievements are remarkable. There is no doubt she experienced episodes of depression and had periods of feeling suicidal before she travelled out to the Crimea, although some authors put this down to her 'enforced idleness' at not being able to pursue her love of nursing. She was very ill with fever in the Crimea and according to Bostridge she contracted brucellosis. In 1861, she additionally developed very bad spinal pain and had to be carried to and from her bed. The paradox is how someone who was so physically ill could pursue such a punishing work schedule and achieve so much from her sick bed. Despite Small's 'jibe' about bipolar disorder, research shows that individuals with bipolar disorder are often highly creative and very productive (Redfield Jamison, 1993). Could bipolar disorder explain her phenomenal output?

Conclusion

Given that Bostridge claims that Florence Nightingale suffered with brucellosis (2008), how can we claim that she is a mental health recovery hero? As discussed above, there is no doubt she suffered with episodes of depression prior to her going to the Crimea where she contracted brucellosis. This does not mean that she did not have a co-morbid mental health problem in her post-Crimea years. Bipolar disorder and PTSD are the two main conditions suggested. If we accept that she had both physical and mental health problems then her productivity and influence on the development of modern nursing and in the improvements in public health, which she helped instigate, are all the more remarkable. In keeping with long-term outcome studies of severe mental illness, which show the majority of individuals go on to make a full recovery (Dorrer, 2006), Florence Nightingale also seems to have made a recovery from her physical and mental ailments in her 60s, and indeed she went on to live until she was 90.

References

Bostridge I (2008) *Florence Nightingale*. London: Penguin.

Campbell A & Jones N (2009) *A World without the Fantastic Five*. London: Time to Change.

Dorrer N (2006) *Evidence of Recovery: The ups and downs of longitudinal outcome research*. Glasgow: Scottish Recovery Network.

Dunbar V (1969) In: F Nightingale (1860) *Notes on Nursing: What it is and what it is not*. New York: Dover Publications.

Jason L, Taylor R, Piloplys S, Stepanek Z & Shlaes J (2002) Evaluating attributions for an illness based upon the name: chronic fatigue syndrome, myalgic encephalopathy and Florence Nightingale disease. *American Journal of Community Psychology* **30** (1) 133–148.

Nightingale F (1860) *Notes on Nursing: What it is and what it is not*. London: Longman.

Nightingale F (1863) *Notes on Hospitals*. London: Longman.

Nightingale F (1871) *Notes on Lying-in Institutions Together with a Proposal for Organising an Institution for Training Midwives and Midwifery Nurses*. London: Longman.

Redfield Jamison K (1993) *Touched with Fire*. New York: Free Press.

Russell WH (1854) Are there no devoted women among us... *The Times*. London: 15th September.

Small H (2010) *Brucellosis and Psychology: Nightingale's depression*. Florence Nightingale: Influence and Inspiration conference. Embley.

Strachey L (2009) *Eminent Victorians*. Oxford: Oxford University Press.

Wisner K, Bostridge M & Mackowiak P (2005) A case of glimmering gloom. *The Pharos* 4–13.

Chapter 3

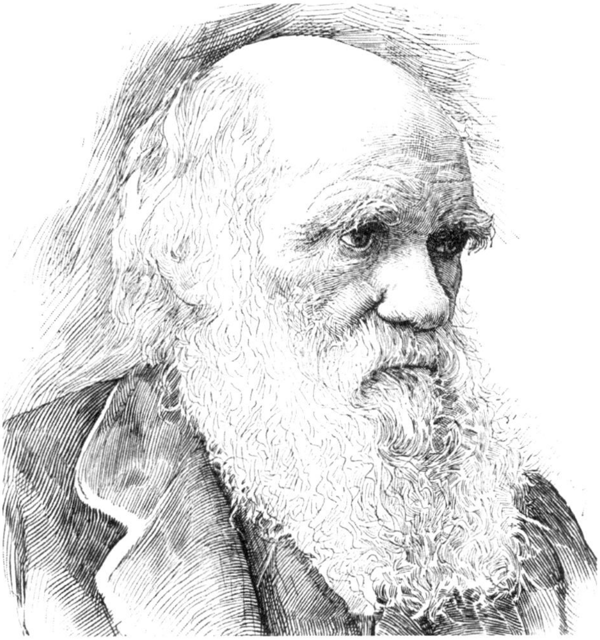

Charles Darwin

Summary

Charles Darwin has been described as one of the greatest scientists of the 19th century, if not *'the greatest scientist who ever lived'* (Bergman, 2004). He expounded the theory of evolution which states, in brief, that life on earth developed, or 'evolved' through the ability of certain species to adapt to their changing environment, while those that could not became extinct (an action which he called natural selection) and that this is a continuous and continuing process. Interest in Darwin's chronic health problems continues to attract the attention of physicians and psychiatrists.

Upbringing and early life

Charles Darwin was born in Shrewsbury on 12th February 1809 to society doctor Robert Darwin (son of Erasmus Darwin, physician and natural philosopher) and his wife Susannah, (daughter of the potter Josiah Wedgwood). His childhood seems to have been unremarkable though firmly bound up with strong Protestant Christianity. He attended schools in Shrewsbury, spending many of his holidays in North Wales where he first developed his taste for natural history and collecting. In 1817 he suffered the loss of his mother when he was just eight, and his father was very authoritarian. In 1825, at the age of 16, he followed the wishes of his father and began to study medicine at Edinburgh University but he did not graduate as he found the subject boring and distressing and was far more interested in natural history. His father, therefore, sent him to Christ's College, Cambridge, hoping to prepare him for an alternative career in the church, but again his interest in natural history predominated. Enthusiastic beetle collecting was encouraged by his cousin, William Darwin Fox, and he attended and was inspired by Professor John Henslow's lectures on botany. It was Henslow who, despite father Robert's objections, set Charles on his career by proposing him as a suitable participant on the Voyage of the Beagle.

Career and achievements

The Voyage of the Beagle

This expedition which set out from Plymouth on 27th December 1831, led by Captain Robert Fitzroy, who was a committed Christian, was commissioned by the Admiralty to survey and chart the coastline of South America. It was intended to last two years but actually lasted five and during that time also visited islands in the Atlantic, Pacific and Indian Oceans, as well as New Zealand and Australia. Darwin, who became chief naturalist, suffered from seasickness throughout the voyage as well as the occasional fever when on land (due to contracting malaria in Santa Fe in 1833 and in 1834 probably from Chagas' disease when he was bitten by Benchuga bugs in the Andes). But he was robust and worked hard, sending reports and specimens back home, especially to Henslow. His work encompassed plants, animals, insects, birds and very importantly, fossils. His first fossil discoveries were made in 1832 and 1833 in Punta Alta, Patagonia, where he found antediluvian animals such as the Toxodon, which is rather like today's hippopotamus, and the Megatherium (a giant sloth), as a result of which he concluded that, although extinct, they closely resembled species still alive. '*This wonderful relationship in the same continent between the dead and the living will, I do not doubt, hereafter throw more light on the appearance of organic beings on earth and their disappearance from it*' (Moorehead, 1969).

In the Andes in 1834, he discovered at 12,000 feet a bed of fossil seashells and a little lower, petrified pine trees surrounded by marine rock deposits, which suggested to him that the mountains had been formed by earthquakes and volcanic eruptions. This view of the instability of the earth in the sense of it changing and developing, not being static, was supported by his investigations in 1836 of coral reefs in Australia, where he noted that here the level had sunk rather than risen. But it was arguably in the Galapagos Islands in September and October 1835 that he made the most important discoveries that would contribute to his view of the evolution of life on this planet. Here there were no mammals but reptiles – tortoises and turtles, iguanas – and land birds of which he found 26 unique species, including finches. What he noticed was that between the different islands, even though they were only 50 or 60 miles apart, the particular species that co-existed differed significantly. Tortoises on different islands had different shells but what was most striking were the differences between the finches whose plumage varied only within limits but whose beaks varied enormously depending, so it seemed, on the food available.

On one island the finches had strong thick beaks for cracking nuts and seeds, on another island the finches had a smaller beak which enabled them to catch insects. On another island their beaks were different again so that they could feed on fruits and flowers. The full implications of this would only become clear to Darwin when he was writing up his findings. He noted: '*Here, both in space and time, we seem to be brought somewhat nearer to that great fact – the mysteries of mysteries – the first appearance of new beings on earth*' (1839).

Subsequent career and the Origin of Species

On the 2nd October 1836, the Beagle dropped anchor at Falmouth and Darwin returned to his family in Shropshire having by this time decided not to pursue a career in the church. From the end of 1836 until 1839 he worked hard, living mainly in London, classifying his specimens and writing up his findings of the Beagle trip, which was published originally as *The Journal of the Voyage of the Beagle* in 1839. He also became Secretary of the Geological Society in London where he became friendly with the geologist Charles Lyell. He was elected a Fellow of the Royal Society in January 1839 and despite some ill-health, he was very active during this period and it was at this time that he realised that a theory of evolution would explain his extraordinary findings. '*July 1837: I opened my first note-book for facts in relation to the origin of species, about which I had long reflected, and never ceased for working for the next twenty years,*' (Neve & Messenger, 2002).

In October 1838 he read Thomas Malthus' *Essay on Population* (1826), which was published 1798, and he recorded in his autobiography '... *it at once struck me that under these circumstances* [i.e. the struggle for existence] *favourable variations would tend to be preserved and unfavourable ones to be destroyed. The result of this would be the formation of a new species. Here, then, I had at last got a theory by which to work,*' (Neve & Messenger, 2002). However, at the time, he was primarily concentrating on writing *The Zoology of the Beagle* (Darwin, 1839), which consisted of five volumes which were published between 1838 and 1843.

Meanwhile, another momentous event in his life had taken place. In January 1839, he married his cousin Emma Wedgwood who was a devout Christian, to whom he became devoted, despite her ambivalent attitude towards, and lack of interest in the minutiae of his work, and she went on to bear him 10 children, seven of whom survived into adulthood.

By 1842, however, Darwin had decided that he had had enough of the stresses of London life and he and his family moved to Down House in Kent, where he led a mentally active but socially reclusive life, rarely venturing beyond the house and its grounds, unless accompanied by his wife. He began to show increasing symptoms of ill health and these included headaches, palpitations, being short of breath, flatulence, nausea and vomiting as well as insomnia, fainting, crying and trembling. However, during the next 14 years he read, researched and experimented prolifically and wrote and published numerous articles on a wide variety of topics in natural history and geology. Then in 1856, on Lyell's advice, and despite his own reservations, because he realised the challenge he was posing to fundamental Christian beliefs and his wife's own deep convictions, he began writing up his views and findings on the transmutation of species for a projected book to be called 'Natural Selection'. However, in June 1858, Darwin received a letter from Alfred Russel Wallace, a naturalist collecting specimens in the Malay Peninsula, which showed that he was coming to the same conclusions as

Darwin himself. On the recommendation of Lyell and Joseph Hooker (fellow botanist and friend), to prevent Wallace stealing Darwin's thunder a paper was presented by them to the Linnaean Society of London on 1st July 1858, giving extracts from the work of both Darwin and Wallace. In November 1859 Darwin's major work *On the Origin of Species by Natural Selection* was finally published. The response was muted at first but slowly the implications began to dawn – not only had God not created the world, entire, complete and unchanging in six days but, although this was a misapprehension, men might actually be descended from apes! This culminated in the historic meeting of the British Association in Oxford in 1860 and the major confrontation that took place between the Bishop of Oxford, Samuel Wilberforce (known as Soapy Sam for his glibness) and TH Huxley, the famous scientist. At first Wilberforce confined himself to attacking Darwin's theories on the basis that they contradicted the literal truth of the Bible but, when he asked Huxley whether it was through his grandfather or his grandmother that he claimed his descent from a monkey, Huxley became incensed and replied that he would not be ashamed to have a monkey for an ancestor but he would be ashamed to be connected with a man who used his great gifts to obscure the truth. Others spoke against Darwin, including his old Captain (now Vice-Admiral) Fitzroy but, although no verbatim account of the debate exists, it seems as though Huxley and Darwin's other supporters, Hooker and Lyell, won the day. Hubbub ensued with ladies fainting and undergraduates cheering. Darwin himself never explicitly denied the existence of God, but was rather an agnostic, and many people nowadays who accept Darwin's theories nevertheless believe in God.

Darwin continued writing for the next 22 years, with his most famous and influential work being the *Descent of Man* (1877), in which he argued that modern man and modern ape had diverged in prehistory from a common line of ancestors and that man's superior faculties had developed thereafter. Interestingly, in the 1860s Darwin's health improved and he made many visits away from Down House, until in December 1881 he began to suffer from heart problems and in April 1882 he died aged 73.

Mental illness aspects

Campbell and Jones commented '*Darwin … experienced anxiety, panic attacks and mental torment that often left him in floods of tears. In modern parlance Darwin had a panic disorder, or severe anxiety,*' (Campbell & Jones, 2009). However, as demonstrated in our portrayal of Florence Nightingale (Wakely

& Carson, 2011), the clinical picture with Charles Darwin is somewhat more complicated than Campbell & Jones' short vignette.

Pickering dates the onset of Darwin's health problems to just before setting sail on the Beagle. '*I was also troubled with palpitations and pains about the heart ... and was convinced I had heart disease,*' (Pickering, 1974) but these could simply have been symptoms of anxiety. Following his marriage in 1839, Darwin began to suffer increasing bouts of illness that interfered with his life and his ability to work. Over time, he started to avoid scientific meetings, society gatherings and dinner parties. He did not participate in the meeting at the Linnaean Society in July 1858, nor in the Oxford Debate of June 1860 and he did not go the publication of the *Origin of Species* in November 1859. He even missed his daughter's wedding and father's funeral as he was 'too ill' to attend. Perhaps most surprisingly, having spent time in Malvern with his dying daughter Annie, Darwin returned to Down House the day before her funeral leaving his sister-in-law and the child's governess to look after the burial (Keynes, 2001).

In his lifetime Darwin consulted more than 20 doctors, including several of the leading specialists of the time. He tried numerous treatments, especially the then fashionable 'water cure' with several trips to various spas, sometimes lasting for months at a time, for his physical symptoms. For these, various explanations have been offered. Pickering (1974) mentions brucellosis, suppressed gout, migraine, diaphragmatic hernia, chronic arsenic poisoning and paroxysmal tachycardia. Adler (1997) suggested Darwin had Chagas' disease and Colp (1997) psychosomatic skin disorder. More recently Campbell & Matthews (2005) have argued that Darwin had systemic lactose intolerance. Even if any, or all, of these may be true, what is clear is that Darwin experienced severe emotional and psychological problems starting with his relationship with his father and his loss of his mother, continuing through his marriage, where he became increasingly dependent on a wife whose religious views he dare not offend (probably not just out of fear but also love and consideration), but eventually had to and, when that internal conflict was resolved with the publication of the *Origin of Species*, he picked up emotionally and psychologically and became more sociable and gregarious.

The balance of the medical evidence is that Darwin had a long-term anxiety disorder (Hubble, 1943; Hubble, 1953; Woodruff, 1965). Hubble (1943) stated, '... *Darwin by his psychoneurosis secretly and passionately nourished his genius; he was protected thus from painful and wasted contacts, escaped from any circumstance which interfered with his work, was rewarded by nights of sleepless suffering which stimulated his restless mind*. This was expanded by Pickering in his book, '*Creative Malady*' in which he states that '... *illness ... can occasionally be of benefit, not only to the victim, but to society,*' a verdict with which we concur.

Appraisal as a recovery hero

While considering the claim that Charles Darwin is a mental health recovery hero, it is important to see the evidence. It is apparent that for 40 years he suffered with a chronic and socially crippling anxiety disorder. This meant that at times he was unable to work for months and even during productive periods when his health was better, he could not work for more than five hours a day (Desmond & Moore, 1991). Anxiety disorders have tended to be neglected in contemporary mental health services with the greater focus being on psychoses (Cordle *et al*, 2011). Few narrative anthologies feature patients suffering with chronic anxiety (Chandler & Hayward, 2009), although there are exceptions (Leibrich, 1999). Yet Darwin continued with his scientific work, despite his mental health problems. He commented, '*My chief enjoyment and sole employment throughout life has been scientific work; and the excitement from such work makes me for the time forget, or drives quite away my daily discomfort,*' (Neve & Messenger, 2002).

Conclusion

Charles Darwin's long-term anxiety disorder was indeed a creative malady. Darwin recognised this himself. '...*I have had ample leisure from not having to earn my own bread. Even ill health, though it has annihilated several years of my life, has saved me from the distractions of society and amusement,*' (Neve & Messenger, 2002). The extreme avoidance resulting from his chronic anxiety meant that Darwin was free to pursue his scientific research to the benefit of posterity.

References

Adler J (1997) *The dueling diagnosis of Darwin. Journal of the American Medical Association* April 23/30, **277** (16) 1275.

Bergman J (2004) Was Charles Darwin psychotic? A study of his mental health. *Impact* **367** i–iv.

Campbell A & Jones N (2009) *A World without the Fantastic Five*. London: Time to Change.

Campbell A & Matthews S (2005) Darwin's illness revealed. *Postgraduate Medical Journal* **81** 248–251.

Chandler R & Hayward M (2009) *Voicing Psychotic Experiences: A reconsideration of recovery and diversity*. Brighton: Pavilion Publishing.

Colp R (1997) The dueling diagnosis of Darwin. *Journal of the American Medical Association* **277** (16) 1275–1276.

Cordle H, Fradgley J, Carson J, Holloway F & Richards P (Eds) (2011) *Psychosis: Stories of recovery and hope*. London: Quay Books.

Darwin C (1839) *Journal of Researches into the Geology and Natural History of the Various Countries visited by HMS Beagle*. London: Henry Colbourn.

Darwin C (1859) *On the Origin of Species by means of Natural Selection or the Preservation of Favoured Races in the Struggle for Life*. London: Murray.

Darwin C (1877) *The Descent of Man: Selection in relation to sex*. London: Murray.

Desmond A & Moore J (1991) *Darwin*. London: Joseph.

Hubble D (1943) Charles Darwin and psychotherapy. *The Lancet*, January 30th 129–133.

Hubble D (1953) The life of the shawl. *The Lancet*, December 26th 1351–1354.

Keynes R (2001) *Creation: The true story of Charles Darwin*. London: John Murray.

Leibrich J (Ed) (1999) *A Gift of Stories*. Dunedin: University of Otago Press.

Maithus T (1826) *An Essay on the Principles of Population*. London: Murray.

Moorehead A (1969) *Darwin and the Beagle*. London: Hamish Hamilton.

Neve M & Messenger S (2002) *Charles Darwin – Autobiographies*. London: Penguin.

Pickering G (1974) *Creative Malady: Illness in the Lives of Charles Darwin, Florence Nightingale, Mary Baker Eddy, Sigmund Freud, Marcel Proust and Elizabeth Barrett Browning*. London: George Allen and Unwin.

Wakely E & Carson J (2011) Historical recovery heroes – Florence Nightingale. *Mental Health and Social Inclusion* **15** (1) 24–28.

Woodruff A (1965) Darwin's health in relation to his voyage to South America. *British Medical Journal* **1** 745–750.

Chapter 4

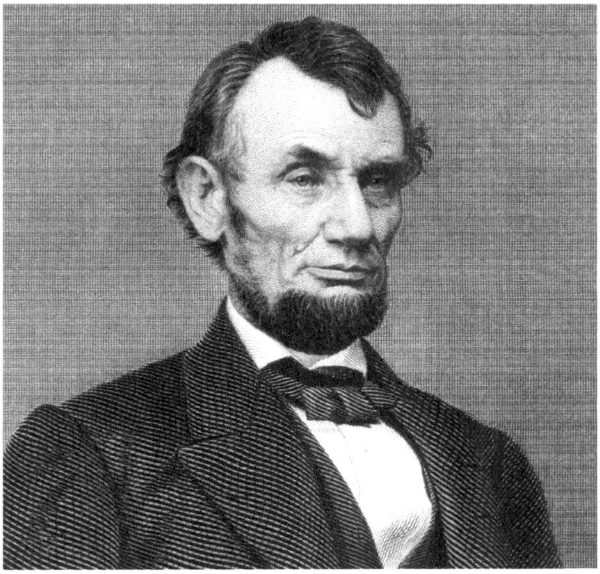

Abraham Lincoln

Summary

Abraham Lincoln is best known for his battle against slavery in the American Civil War, but what is less well known is his lifelong internal battle with a major depressive illness. Yet as one expert points out what stands out about Lincoln is not his psychological weakness, but his remarkable strength.

Upbringing and early life

Abraham Lincoln was born in a one-room log cabin in Kentucky on 12th February 1809, as the second child of Thomas and Nancy Lincoln. His childhood was not an easy one because, although not as poor as his place of birth might suggest, his family had its ups and downs and their livelihood lay in farming. His father was reputedly a difficult and moody man who did not believe in education beyond the basics for his children. Consequently young Abe was largely self-taught and was considered lazy because he liked reading although he did all that he was required to do on the family farms, at first in Kentucky, then Indiana and, finally, Illinois and he became an expert in building rail fences.

In 1818, when he was nine, his mother died of 'milk-sickness' and before that a younger brother died in infancy in 1812. His older sister Sarah to whom he was very close died in childbirth in 1828. However, one must remember that such early deaths were not infrequent at the time, and he was generally considered to be a gregarious and well-liked child. Thomas, his father, to whom he was not close, was remarried in 1819 to Sarah Johnston, a stepmother of whom Abe became very fond and whom he called 'mother'. In 1831 Lincoln left the family home and settled in New Salem, Illinois, where he lived until he moved in 1837 to Springfield, the new state capital of Illinois, where he remained until he moved to Washington when he became President in 1861.

During this period he qualified as a lawyer, and became interested and involved in politics and also formed a number of romantic attachments. The first, according to popular accounts, although disputed by Shenk (2006) was to Ann Rutledge who died in August 1835. What is certainly clear is that it was at this time that for whatever reason Lincoln suffered his first breakdown and contemplated suicide. '[Lincoln] *told me that he felt like committing suicide often'* (mentor Graham quoted in Shenk, 2006) and *'Mr Lincoln's friends ... were compelled to keep watch...'* (Shenk, 2006).

In 1836–1837 he became involved with and proposed to Mary Owens, who turned him down, and his melancholy was apparent. *'He was a sad looking man, gloomy and melancholic,'* (William Herndon quoted in Shenk, 2006). Then in 1839 he met and proposed to Mary Todd but the engagement was broken off in January 1841 when he had his second breakdown and again, his friends feared suicide. However, in November 1842, the pair finally married, although when preparing for the occasion and asked where he was going, Lincoln replied *'To Hell, I suppose'*, (quoted in Shenk, 2006). The marriage was certainly not an easy one as Mary herself was mentally unstable, but it produced four sons to whom Lincoln was devoted, although only one survived him. The deaths of the other three were deeply felt tragedies for both parents and in 1875, Robert, the eldest, had his mother committed to an asylum. However, it would be an over-simplification to attribute Lincoln's famed '*melancholy*' to romantic failures alone, as much else was going on and 1841 was a critical year in his professional and political life, during which he told his friend, Joshua Speed, that '*he had an "irrepressible desire" to accomplish something while he lived,*' (Shenk, 2006).

Career and achievements

Early career

Lincoln's life for the next 19 years after his marriage was largely played out in Springfield where he became a respected figure. In 1834 he had taken up his first political post as a member of the Illinois General Assembly and in 1836 he qualified as a lawyer, in which career he was an assiduous practitioner and a recognised success. In politics he moved from the local to the national stage becoming a Congressman for Illinois from 1846 to 1849 but never, as he had hoped, a Senator. However, all that changed when, on 6th November 1860, as leader of the newly formed Republican Party and the 'rail' candidate (a reference to his humble origins) he was elected 16th President of the United States.

Presidency

Lincoln took office on 4th March 1861 but between his election and his inauguration cataclysmic events had taken place: seven states, South Carolina, Mississippi, Florida, Alabama, Georgia, Louisiana and Texas (later to be joined by four others: Virginia, North Carolina, Tennessee and Arkansas) had seceded from the 'union' of the United States to form the Confederate States or Confederacy under their own President, Jefferson Davis, over the issue of slavery.

This issue was a complex one and although retrospectively usually couched in ideological/idealistic terms, at the time it was often more a matter of political and economic expediency. By 1861 the original 13 states had expanded to 34, with most of the Western part of the country being known as territories and not yet fully incorporated as states of the union. The 18 northern states were going through an industrial revolution and their economy was dependent on free wage labour, of which they needed more. This could be supplied by freed slaves. The southern states depended on the cotton and tobacco plantations for their prosperity on which they employed bond or slave labour. In order to increase their labour force, they wanted the extension of slavery into any newly formed states, something which Lincoln had always opposed. In brief, the North was against slavery and the South was in favour of it.

In 1858 he made an impassioned speech at Quincy, Illinois: '*We have in this nation the element of domestic slavery ... we think it is a moral, a social and a political wrong ... We will deal with it as any other wrong, insofar as we can prevent it growing any larger, and so deal with it that in the run of time there may be some promise of an end to it.*'

However, at this point he was not an out and out abolitionist. This is not to say that there were no abolitionists, because there were. In fact the first action of what would later become a full-blown civil war took place in 1859 when John Brown, a fanatical abolitionist with 18 supporters seized the government arsenal at Harper's Ferry, Virginia, and issued a proclamation in an attempt to encourage a slave rebellion. The attempt failed and John Brown was hanged, though in the words of the song, '*his soul goes marching on*'. So the spectrum of opinion ranged from retention and extension of slavery through the middle ground of allowing existing slavery but not extending it, to complete abolition of the practice. And it had long been a festering matter of debate.

By the time he arrived at the White House, therefore Lincoln faced a nation in turmoil. He said to his election campaigners, '*Well, boys, your troubles are over, but mine have just begun!*' (Shenk, 2006). This was an indication of his wry sense of humour and indeed he was renowned as an excellent and witty raconteur, another side to this melancholic and complex man. In his inaugural address of 4th March 1861, he attempted to avoid conflict by saying he had no intention '*to interfere with the institution of slavery in the states where it exists. I believe I have no lawful right to do so*'. But the confederates were not mollified and the Civil War began when they attacked the government Fort Sumter in Charleston, Virginia, on 12th April 1861.

This chapter is not long enough for a detailed account of the military operations of the conflict between North and South. Lincoln was determined above all else to preserve the union and to win back the Confederate States. The North comprised 23 states and 22,000,000 people, while the Confederacy was made up of only 11 states and 9,000,000 people (including 3,500,000 slaves). Yet, despite this superiority in numbers and resources, it took four years of bitter and bloody battles with enormous losses on both sides, until on the 9th April 1865 the Confederates under General Robert E Lee surrendered to northern General Ulysses S Grant at Appomattox Court House in Virginia.

In this story, the year 1863 was a momentous year as it marked the turning point in the war when the Confederates were defeated on 3rd July at the Battle of Gettysburg and, what is possibly more important, having been reflecting on it for two years, Lincoln finally came out against slavery on 1st January when he issued his Emancipation Proclamation freeing all slaves in lands held by the confederates. To celebrate, on 9th November, Lincoln delivered his famous Gettysburg Address on the site of the battle:

'Four score and seven years ago our fathers brought forth on this continent a new nation, conceived in liberty and dedicated to the proposition that all men are created equal. Now we are engaged in a great civil war, testing whether that nation, or any nation so conceived and so dedicated, can long endure. We are met on a great battlefield of that war. We have come to dedicate a portion of that field as a final resting place for those who here gave their lives that that nation might live. It is altogether fitting and proper that we should do this. But, in a larger sense, we cannot dedicate, we cannot consecrate, we cannot hallow this ground. The brave men, living and dead, who struggled here have consecrated it, far above our poor power to add or detract. The world will little note, nor long remember, what we say here but it can never forget what they did here. It is for us the living, rather, to be dedicated here to the unfinished work which they who fought here have thus far so nobly advanced. It is rather for us to be here dedicated to the great task remaining before us, that from these honoured dead we take increased devotion to that cause for which they gave the last full measure of devotion, that we here highly resolve that these dead shall not have died in vain, that this nation, under God, shall have a new birth of freedom and that government of the people, by the people, for the people, shall not perish from the earth.'

The war was over on 9th April 1865 but the President was only able to savour the sweet taste of victory for five days as on 14th April he was shot in the head at Ford's Theatre by John Wilkes Booth, and he died the following day.

Achievement

Abraham Lincoln preserved the union of the United States and freed the slaves. Without his presidency the subsequent history not only of America but of the world would have been very different. However it took another hundred years for black Americans to achieve legal equality with white citizens through the passing of the Civil Rights Act in 1964 and the Voting Rights Act in 1965. This came about as a result of the rise of the Civil Rights Movement under the leadership of Martin Luther King, which was prompted by several events that drew attention to the inequalities that faced black Americans and the resistance they posed. The story of Rosa Parks who refused to give up her seat to a white person on a bus in Montgomery, Alabama, in 1955 was the one of the incidents covered by the media, which drew attention to the cause. In 1957 the media covered the controversy in Little Rock, Arkansas, where nine black children gained admission to an all white high school.

The United States now has its first non-white President in Barack Obama who came to office just weeks before the 200th anniversary of the birth of Abraham Lincoln. Obama feels a sense of kinship with Lincoln as they both represented Illinois and he paid tribute to him in his Inaugural Address of 20th January 2009.

Mental illness aspects

Unlike two of our other historical recovery heroes, Florence Nightingale and Charles Darwin, who had possible physical causes for their problems, Abraham Lincoln clearly suffered from a recurrent depressive illness. It is also of note that while our four other historical figures had only short journal papers written about their mental health problems, there have been two books written just on Lincoln's mental health (Burlingame, 1997; Shenk, 2006).

Shenk's account of Lincoln's mental health problems is the more comprehensive. He tries to answer three main questions. First, did Lincoln have a clinical depression? Second, what kind of treatment did he undergo? Third, how did melancholy contribute to his work as a public figure?

1. Did Lincoln have a clinical depression?

Henry Witney declared, '*No element of Mr Lincoln's character was so marked, obvious, and ingrained as his mysterious and profound melancholy*', (Shenk, 2006). His law partner William Herndon said, '*His melancholy, dripped from him as he walked,*' (Shenk, 2006). Albert Beveridge concluded that the last decade and a half of Lincoln's life was dominated, '*... by a sadness so profound that the depths of it cannot be* *sounded or estimated by normal minds,'* (Burlingame, 1997). Lincoln also had a family history of depression. As pointed out earlier, he experienced significant loss in his childhood. His only brother died in infancy, and his mother died when he was nine. The one constant in his early life was his sister Sarah, yet she died after giving birth when he was 19. It was seven years later following the death of his friend, Anna Rutledge, that he experienced his first serious episode of depression. *'The subsequent events of Lincoln's life that plunged him into Stygian gloom, had such power because they awakened memories of the painful losses he suffered as a youth'* (Burlingame, 1997).

Paradoxically, Shenk points out, *'Lincoln's melancholy ... seems to have helped him thrive ... his moods constantly provoked empathy, assistance and admiration'* (Shenk, 2006). William Butler tried to cheer Lincoln up, and finding that he was unable to, he went and paid some of his debts, took his clothes home so his wife could wash them, and insisted Lincoln come and live with them. Lincoln experienced another depressive episode following the collapse of his plans to transform the state economy through his internal improvements scheme. He declared at the time, *'I am now the most miserable man living,'* (Shenk, 2006). He was then aged 32.

2. What kind of treatment did he undergo?

After his second episode of clinical depression, Lincoln was treated by a Dr Henry, *'who put him to bed and kept him isolated. But if Dr Henry followed the standard course of treatment with Lincoln, he would have bled him, purged him and puked him, starved him, dosed him with mercury and pepper, rubbed him with mustard and plunged him in cold water,'* (Shenk, 2006). Lincoln himself believed there were three things that could affect those of a nervous disposition. These were bad weather, isolation or idleness and stressful events.

Lincoln seems to have used two main strategies to cope with his depressive illness. The first was telling jokes and stories. He studiously collected new material to share with others and this was something he developed early in his life. *'By the time he was a teenager, grown men would flock around him, eager to hear his jokes and stories. He was well liked,'* (Shenk, 2006). The other main strategy he adopted was to read, recite and compose poetry that dwelled on the themes of death, despair and human futility.

3. How did melancholy contribute to his life as public figure?

Interestingly, and unlike contemporary attitudes to mental illness, Lincoln's depression did not seem to matter to people of that time. Indeed one politician raised the issue not to question Lincoln's fitness for office, but to show how he had triumphed over difficulty. At the outset of the Civil War, Shenk (2006) comments, '*After a lifetime of inner turmoil, Lincoln had the experience and judgement to look trouble straight in the eye*'. Again he noted, '*... a tendency to depressive realism – a temperamental inclination to see and prepare for the worst, gave* [Lincoln] *an advantage.*'

Appraisal as a recovery hero

Gordon McManus' definition of recovery as, '*coping with your illness and having a meaningful life,*' (see Chapter 15) applies to Lincoln, as it does to all five of our historical recovery heroes. Each of these major historical figures had to cope with a long-term mental health problem, yet each was able to lead not just a meaningful life but a life which profoundly affected the world in which they lived. Shenk explains this paradox in discussing Lincoln's life, '*... Lincoln also meets the surgeon general's criteria for mental health; the successful performance of mental function, resulting in productive activities, fulfilling relationships with other people, and the ability to adapt and change and cope with adversity,*' (Shenk, 2006).

In terms of living a meaningful life, Lincoln commented to his old friend Joshua Speed, '*... die when I may, I want it said of me by those who know me best ... that I always plucked a thistle and planted a flower when I thought a flower would grow,*' (Burlingame, 1997). Again he said to Speed, '*I am not afraid, and would be more than willing to die. But I have an irrepressible desire to live till I can be assured that the world is a little better for my having lived in it,*' (Burlingame, 1997).

Lincoln's coping techniques have already been commented on. '*To relieve the gloom, Lincoln resorted to humour; his legendary storytelling and joking were essential to his mental balance ... I have hours of depression, which must be unbent ... You know I am not a man of very hopeful temperament,*' (Burlingame, 1997). In a poem he wrote in 1846, '*My childhood home I see again,*' Lincoln is obsessed with '*loved ones lost ... and half of all are dead*'. He especially admired Oliver Wendell Holmes' *The Last Leaf*. He was fondest of the following stanza:

The mossy marbles rest
On lips that he has pressed
In their bloom;
And the names he loved to hear
Have been carved for many a year
On the tomb.

(Burlingame, 1997)

Conclusion

Burlingame is in no doubt that Lincoln's inner life profoundly affected his outer life in a positive manner. '*My assessment of the Lincoln marital woes stresses the ways in which they taught Lincoln how to cope with difficult people, helped to fuel his ambition, and led him to invest much of his emotional capital in his political career,*' (1997). His whole life shows how even though he suffered with a long-term recurrent depressive illness Lincoln was still able to become '*arguably America's greatest president,*' (Campbell & Jones, 2009).

References

Burlingame M (1997) *The Inner World of Abraham Lincoln*. Chicago: University of Illinois Press.

Campbell A & Jones (2009) *A World Without the Fantastic Five*. London: Time to Change.

Shenk J (2006) *Lincoln's Melancholy: How depression challenged a president and fuelled his greatness*. New York: Houghton Mifflin.

Chapter 5

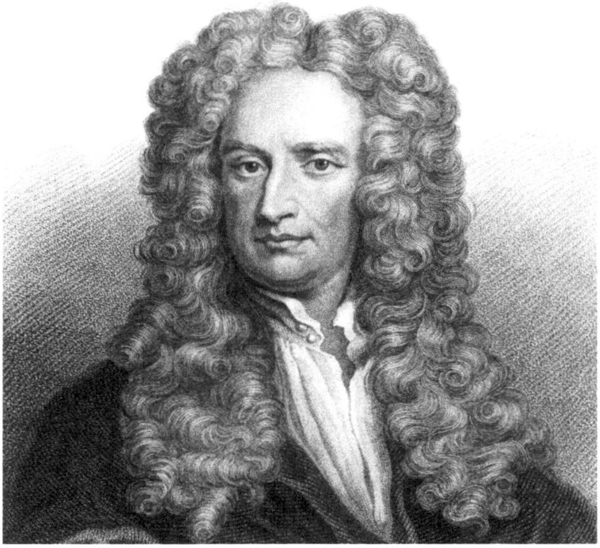

Isaac Newton

Summary

Isaac Newton has been described as the pioneer and father of modern science, who made major contributions to the fields of physics, mathematics and astronomy. Yet, he devoted more time to the study of theology and alchemy. He developed mental health problems during his time at Cambridge and in 1693 he experienced a 'psychotic' breakdown, which some authors feel was due to mercury poisoning. It seems more likely that this was due to recurrent depression or even that he may have had bipolar disorder.

Early life and upbringing

The circumstances of Isaac Newton's birth were less than auspicious as he was born prematurely and posthumously into a yeoman family in Woolsthorpe, Lincolnshire on Christmas Day 1642. Later, he himself would consider the date significant. His mother, Hannah, remarried in 1646 when he was just three, and she left her son in the care of his grandparents with whom there is no record of any affection; indeed his grandfather left him out of his will. In 1653, after the death of her second husband Hannah returned to him but with three half-siblings in tow. In 1654, Isaac was sent to King's School, Grantham, and lodged with the local apothecary, Mr Clark and his family where he was not very happy. Newton wrote at the time of his experiences, '*A little fellow; my poore help; hee is paile; there is no room for me to sit; – in the top of the house – in the bottom of hell; what imployment is he fit for? What is he good for? I will make an end. I cannot but weepe, I do not not know what to doe,*' (Gleick, 2003).

He wasn't particularly interested in the school's classical curriculum but spent a lot of time in the apothecary's shop experimenting with chemicals, which may have triggered his future interest in alchemy and in building working models, for example, of a local windmill – a trigger for his interest in mechanics. He didn't get on with other children but after an encounter with a bully and winning the physical fight, he decided to prove his worth by achieving academically. Although maths and science were not part of the curriculum (which makes Newton's future achievements all the more remarkable), learning Latin was compulsory. Knowledge of Latin later enabled Newton to communicate with other European scholars as at the time, this was the language of scientific communication. Indeed, most of Newton's own works were originally written in Latin.

However, in 1659 his mother decided to remove him from school to manage the family estate in which he showed not the slightest interest, and in 1660 Henry Stokes, the headmaster of the grammar school persuaded her to send him back to school. The family servants were delighted saying that he was '*fit for nothing but the Versity*,' (Stukeley cited in White, 1997).

In 1661, Isaac duly went up to Trinity College, Cambridge, as a subsizar (the lowliest of students whose tasks included emptying the chamber pots of fellows) to study natural philosophy, where he came under the influence of Isaac Barrow. Barrow became the first Lucasian Professor of Mathematics in 1663 (a post now held by Professor Stephen Hawking) and was instrumental in getting him elected to a scholarship in 1664, which was vital both to improving his social standing and getting him a fellowship later. In 1665 Isaac Newton gained his BA, and Stukeley is quoted saying: '*When Sir Isaac stood for his Bachelor of Arts degree, he was put in second posing, or lost his groats, as they call it, which is looked upon as disgraceful,*' (White, 1997). In more modern parlance, he did poorly in his viva examination. In the same year the plague hit Cambridge and closed down the university. Newton went home to Woolsthorpe for the next two years where he completed his work on the calculus, four years after arriving at Cambridge with no previous history of studying maths. He also studied optics as well as mechanics and motion and began his work on gravity. The famous story of the apple (which is when Newton saw the apple fall from the tree and it made him consider the principle of gravity) dates from this time. In effect, he taught himself through his intellectual curiosity and this was one of the most productive periods of his life. On his return to Cambridge in March 1667 he was elected a Fellow of Trinity. In 1668 he passed his MA and in October 1669 he was appointed Lucasian Professor of Mathematics on the resignation of Barrow. It had taken Newton only eight years to make the transition from fresher to professor.

Cambridge years

The next 30 years of Newton's life were spent in Cambridge working on his scientific interests, which included physics, maths and astronomy, and he often gave the occasional mandatory lecture to an empty room as the students were unable to grasp his ideas. Indeed, on the publication of his most famous work *Philosophiae Naturalis Principia Mathematica (Mathematical Principles of Natural Philosophy*), a student commented on passing Newton in the street, '*There goes the man that writt a book that neither he nor anybody else understands!*' (Westfall, 1993).

His years at Cambridge were solitary and lonely and he concentrated so hard on his work that he frequently forgot to eat. In the 1670s he was working and lecturing on optics and he constructed a reflecting telescope, which was demonstrated in 1671 to the Royal Society of which he was elected a Fellow in 1672 and later in 1703 to become President. Some of his ideas were published in the *Philosophical Transactions of the Royal Society* in 1672, which led to a quarrel with the scientist Robert Hooke that was to last for 30 years. It was in a reply to Hooke that he stated, '*If I have seen further, it is by standing on ye shoulders of giants,*' (Westfall, 1993).

While sounding complimentary to Hooke and modest about himself, it was a coded insult as Hooke was short in stature. But, on the whole, he was very secretive about his work and suspicious of sharing his knowledge and it was not until 1704 that he finally published his *Opticks* (1721), expounding his theories of colour and light. Similarly, although he was working on mechanics and gravitation and writing in notebooks for some 20 years, it was only in 1687 that his magnum opus *The Principia* (1687) (referred to above) was published, in which he presented his three laws of motion and his theory of universal gravitation. Meanwhile he was also experimenting in alchemy, a dangerous and forbidden subject but one that he thought superior to ordinary chemistry because it embraced a spiritual element, and writing on Christian theology and the chronology and prophecies of the Bible. His religious views were unorthodox because, although he was a firm believer in God the Father as omnipotent, omniscient and omnipresent, he denied the doctrine of the Trinity (ironical for one who made his living from Trinity College) and, until his deathbed, when he refused the sacrament, he kept them largely to himself.

In order to remain at Cambridge he should have been ordained into the Anglican Church but, with help from Barrow, in 1675 he got a dispensation from King Charles II allowing him to continue without ordination. It was through alchemy that in 1689 he met Nicolas Fatio de Duillier, a Swiss mathematician, with whom he had an intense relationship bordering on infatuation until it came to an abrupt end in 1693. Personal relationships were always difficult for Newton, especially as he had no capacity for forgiveness, and he quarrelled not only with Hooke (see above) but also famously with Gottfried Leibniz over which of them had first discovered the calculus (a dispute that lasted 40 years) and over a period of years, with Sir John Flamsteed, the Astronomer Royal. To try and resolve the question of priority with Leibniz, he set up a commission at the Royal Society to examine all the documentation on the calculus dispute. Newton declared somewhat self-righteously that, '*No man is a witness in his own cause,*' (Gleick, 2003).

It was he who wrote the report on the matter and he clearly found evidence in his own favour. Newton did however have some influential friends, including the diarist Samuel Pepys and the philosopher John Locke, and it was two paranoid and delusional letters written to them in September 1693 that indicated the state of Newton's mental health and the psychotic breakdown that he was suffering. The acute period of his illness was, fortunately, short-lived and also fortunately, his career was about to take another direction, thanks to his friends in high places.

Old age

In 1696 Newton was appointed Warden, then in 1700 Master of the Royal Mint in London. He left Cambridge forever and spent the last 30 years of his life as an administrator and civil servant overseeing the recoinage, and pursuing counterfeiters; as a very public figure this was a sea change from his Cambridge days. In 1796 his niece, Catherine Barton (later to become Catherine Conduitt, wife of John Conduitt who would succeed Newton as Master of the Mint and write a biography of him), became his housekeeper and from then on he became much more hospitable, enjoying the society of the great and the good. But many of his old characteristics were still in evidence, as can be seen from his relentless and vindictive pursuit of the arch-counterfeiter, William Chaloner, whom he brought to the gallows in 1699 – a story brilliantly retold in *Newton and the Counterfeiters* (Levenson, 2009).

In his work at the Mint, Newton was extremely thorough, efficient and hardworking, and as usual he quickly grasped the principles of economics although, ironically, he was a victim of the South Sea Bubble in 1720, a speculative, over-subscribed and catastrophically unsuccessful financial venture of that time. For once his acquisitiveness overcoming careful judgement. He was knighted by Queen Anne in 1705 and died a grand old man in 1727, and was buried in Westminster Abbey. The tribute on his monument reads, '*Let mortals rejoice that there has existed such and so great an ornament to the human race.*'

Or as Alexander Pope (1683–1744) put it both grandiloquently and somewhat facetiously in his intended epitaph:

'*Nature and Nature's laws lay hid in Night:*
God said "Let Newton be!" and all was Light!'

Achievements

Sir Isaac Newton was knighted for public service but his achievements and legacy lie in science. However, it was not only his ideas that paved the way for modern science (just as his mechanics paved the way for the industrial revolution) but also his methods. He was not just satisfied with theories and hypotheses ('hypotheses non fingo') (second edition of *The Principia*, 1713): they had to be demonstrable, hence his emphasis on induction from experimentation (even to the extent of forcing a bodkin behind his eyeball and tasting the results of his alchemical experiments). Newton's focus on conducting rigorous experiments can be seen as the beginning of modern scientific methods. This can be noted in his quotation: '*Amicus Plato, Amicus Aristotles, magis amica veritas.*' Translated this means: '*Plato and Aristotle are my friends but my greater friend is Truth,*' (quoted in Westfall, 1993). At the time university education at Cambridge was based on the study Greek philosophers. Newton was never satisfied with their theories, which were not based on careful experimentation.

Mental illness aspects

At the outset it is perhaps wise to heed Anthony Storr's (1985) advice, '*In a subject in which so much is controversial, it behoves both the psychiatrist and the historian to be modest in their claims to psychological understanding*'.

There are three aspects which we will address with respect to Newton's mental health. First, we will look at his breakdown of 1693; second, we will look at his childhood; and third, we will consider personality issues.

The bulk of the literature on Newton's mental illness centres on his breakdown in 1693. A number of authors have suggested his breakdown was caused by exposure to mercury through his alchemical experiments (Spivack & Epstein, 2001; Keynes, 1980, 2008). Broad (1981) reports that Newton tasted the results of his experiments on at least 108 occasions, and Ditchburn (1980) provides the most comprehensive review of the mercury hypothesis. He starts by describing the symptoms of Newton's 'psychosis' and claims evidence of this 'psychosis' (see also Jeste *et al*, 2000) comes largely from correspondence, such as a letter to Pepys where Newton said, '*I must withdraw from your acquaintance, and see neither you or any of my friends anymore*'. The same day he wrote to Locke and stated, '*You have attempted to embroil me with women*'. Yet, some two weeks later, following a visit from Millington, a mutual friend of Pepys and Newton's, told Pepys that Newton had realised that he had written a very odd letter while he was not well. Millington feared he was, '... *under some small degree of melancholy,*' (Ditchburn, 1980).

Ditchburn summarises Newton's symptoms thus:

1. He had suffered with insomnia for at least a year.
2. He was depressed and wanted to withdraw from the few close friends he had.

3. He had a loss of appetite.
4. For a period he suffered delusions that his friends were against him.

Ditchburn (1980) goes on to show that Newton did not show any of the classic symptoms of mercurialism; he had no pains in his mouth, his writing showed no signs of tremor and he had no excitability. He concludes that Newton's symptoms were more consistent with depression.

Lieb & Hershman (1983) having also reviewed and dismissed the evidence for mercurialism as having caused Newton's breakdown, go on to suggest that his crisis of 1693 was an exacerbation of a manic depressive illness. They argue that Newton had a previous breakdown in 1664, when a period of overwork and insomnia were followed by a depressive episode. In the next two years Newton achieved his highest level of creativity, which they feel points to a period of hypomania. Then, as we see it, the completion of *The Principia* in 1687 was preceded by 18 months of excitement and astonishing productivity, after which he may have experienced significant feelings of deflation. These feelings may have been exacerbated by the breakup of the relationship with Fatio, in which there may have been an element of repressed homosexuality (a thesis supported by the absence of a paternal role model, his ambivalent relationship with his mother and the lack of evidence of any emotional or sexual relationships with other women), which, in a man so puritanically religious as he would have led to agonies of guilt. Also the fact that not only was his alchemy work not leading anywhere but was actually causing him another irreconcilable emotional conflict and the realisation that his most creative days were probably now behind him, all of which precipitated a crisis. Lieb & Hershman conclude that Newton remained complex, paradoxical and manic depressive to the end.

The second aspect of Newton's mental health that needs to be commented on is his early upbringing. As pointed out earlier, his mother left Newton with his maternal grandparents at the age of three and did not return until eight years later. His father died three months before he was born and Westfall comments, '*Isaac's boyhood appears to have been lonely. He formed no bond with any of his numerous relations that can be traced in his later life. The lonely boyhood was the first chapter in a long career of isolation*' (Westfall, 1993). While it has been noted that Newton was close to his mother (Broad, 1981), Westfall (1993) points out that in the 12 years after his return to Cambridge following the plague, he paid a maximum of only six visits to Woolsthorpe to see his mother. He observes, '*More vigorous displays of filial affection have been recorded*'. Storr (1985) comments that he feels Newton's childhood was classically traumatic and that it must have affected his later personality.

The third aspect of Newton's mental health is his personality. White (1997) suggests that Newton was '... *far more twisted and convoluted than historians of science would have us believe*'. James (2003) in a review of very eminent scientists notes that Professor Simon Baron Cohen has diagnosed both Newton and Einstein as having Asperger's syndrome. He reports that Newton was '... *unable to form intimate friendships. Morbidly suspicious and secretive, he was subject to peevish outbreaks of ill temper ... On such occasions he stooped to regrettable acts which involved him in a succession of painful controversies that plagued his life, robbed him of the just fruits of his work and disheartened his sincere admirers.*' Storr (1985) presents a detailed perspective on Newton's personality. Among other characteristics, he notes that the counterfeiters that Newton pursued when Warden of the Mint served the same function for him as did Hitler for Churchill. They gave him a channel for his aggressive feelings. White (1997) suggests that there was also a grandiose and somewhat delusional nature to Newton's personality, '*Would it be unreasonable to suggest that he* [Newton] *wanted to identify himself with Christ? After all was he not the only child of a dead father, born on Christmas Day and (so he believed) possessed of unparalleled ability and unique talents?*'

Appraisal as a recovery hero

Newton not only recovered from his breakdown in 1693 but he decided to leave Cambridge and give up the career of a scientist for that of an administrator, when he became Warden then Master of the Mint. His knowledge of metallurgy from his alchemical experiments helped him with the recoinage, and his scientific approach to tackling problems enabled him to become successful in this new field. His life also shows that sometimes a genius can emerge from a traumatic background. He never knew his father. His mother left him from the age of three to 11. Despite these losses he went on to become one of the greatest scientists to have lived. His social isolation and his complete dedication also helped him achieve his breakthroughs. As Storr (1985) observes: '... *if intense periods of concentration over long periods are required to attain fundamental insights, the family man is at a disadvantage.*'

Conclusion

Studying Isaac Newton's mind seems almost as complex as many of the mysteries his scientific work tried to unravel. Indeed, Jeste and colleagues (2000) caution, '*The trail of evidence is probably too cold for us to ever know definitively what his illness was or what caused it.*'

There is no doubt that his upbringing was traumatic; and that he had serious personality difficulties and that he experienced at least two episodes of mental breakdown. His isolation, single mindedness and dedication helped contribute to his greatness. It is perhaps fitting to end this brief review with one of Newton's more modest assessments of his work.
'*I do not know what I may appear to the world, but to myself I seem to have been like a boy, playing on the sea shore and diverting myself in now and then finding a smoother pebble or a prettier shell than ordinary, while the great ocean of truth lay all undiscovered before me,*' (White, 1997).

References

Broad W (1981) Sir Isaac Newton: mad as a hatter. *Science* **213** 1341–1344.

Ditchburn R (1980) Newton's illness of 1692–1693. *Notes and Proceedings of the Royal Society of London* **35** (1) 1–16.

Gleick J (2003) *Isaac Newton*. London: Fourth Estate.

James I (2003) Singular scientists. *Journal of the Royal Society of Medicine* **96** 36–39.

Jeste D, Harless K & Palmer B (2000) Chronic late onset schizophrenia like psychosis that remitted: revisiting Newton's psychosis. *American Journal of Psychiatry* **157** (3) 444–449.

Keynes M (1980) Sir Isaac Newton and his madness of 1692–1693. *The Lancet* **529–530**.

Keynes M (2008) Balancing Newton's mind: his singular behaviour and his madness of 1692–1693. *Notes and Records of the Royal Society* **62** 289–300.

Levenson T (2009) *Newton and the Counterfeiters*. London: Faber.

Lieb J & Hershman D (1983) Isaac Newton: mercury poisoning or manic depression? *The Lancet* **24–31**, 1479–1480.

Newton I (1687) *The Principia: Mathematical principles of natural philosophy*. London: William Dawson.

Newton I (1721) *Opticks: Or a treatise on the reflections, inflections and colours of light*. London: Bell.

Spivack M & Epstein M (2001) Newton's psychosis. *American Journal of Psychiatry* **158** (5) 821–822.

Storr A (1985) Isaac Newton. *British Medical Journal* **29** 1779–1784.

Westfall R (1993) *The Life of Isaac Newton*. Cambridge: Cambridge University Press.

White M (1997) *Isaac Newton: The last sorcerer*. London: Fourth Estate.

Part 2: Contemporary Recovery Heroes

Chapter 6

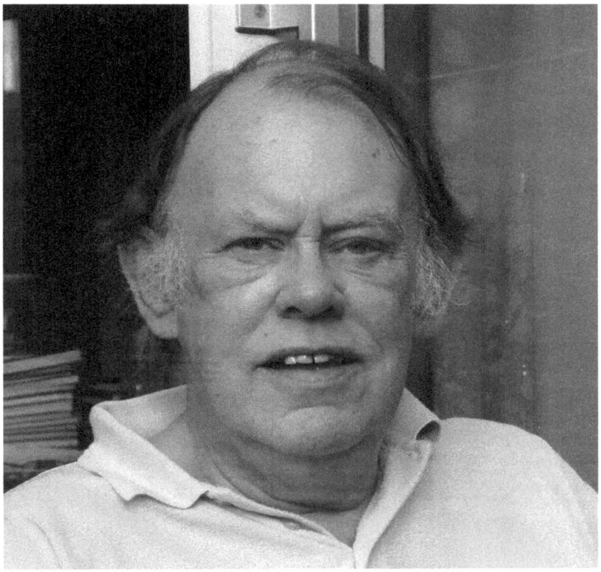

Peter Chadwick

Summary

Peter had a psychotic episode in 1979 that led to a serious suicide attempt and a hospital admission. He was later to use his understanding of his own episode to develop his theories of psychosis. He has called this the peer professional approach, and few people have written as much on psychology and psychosis.

Peter in his own words

One of the questions that has always preoccupied me in recent decades is, 'does a psychotic episode mean anything?' And if it does, does it help to delve into these things? Neither the bio-medical model of psychiatry nor the usual 'recovery' models deal with this issue, which is more the preserve of existential and psychoanalytic thought on the topic of psychosis.

I personally believe that psychotic episodes and psychotic symptoms do have meaning and hence that they possess narrative sense. They are not just '*empty speech acts*' from a diseased brain as Berrios (1991) suggests. Unresolved guilt and shame had a great deal to do with my own crisis in 1979. Transvestism and bisexuality were my sins in the 1970s. There wasn't the light hearted attitude to such ways of being back then that there is now. Attitudes made me feel like I ought to pay for my transgressions with suffering. Also my relationship with my mother who had died in 1971 was incredibly troubled. We rowed endlessly and I even felt in 1979 that she was reaching out from beyond the grave in revenge to punish me for not being a '*good enough son*'. My delusions and occasional hallucinations were pretty well modelled on the treatment I had received from a bullying ring at school and from 'scandal mongers' in the community.

Delving into the origin of my crisis made me realise what kind of people had provoked it – and hence what kind of people to have nothing to do with in the future. By mixing with people congruent with my temperament and by doing work that more fully expressed my style of being – as well as marrying a fully accepting woman, I was able to avoid going down roads in my life that would lead to similar problems again. Indeed, I have had no 'relapses' and even my 'alternative sexuality' changed back to straight sex as I found that my femininity was more fully expressed in the kind of teaching I did than in cross-dressing. Hence it turned out that enquiring into meanings and causes was indeed vitally helpful for recovery, not just pondering 'how to get out of it'.

My episode was over 30 years ago and it is true that I have felt a lot better since the crisis than I did before, when I lived a very anguished and unsettled life. A tiny amount of haloperidol has made me feel more like my real self than I felt before, as it seemed to take away barriers to the emergence of the real self rather than turning me into someone I'm not.

The creative life has also been a great antidote to madness. In many ways creative writing has healed my mind by externalising what is within and making it useful via addressing the content to more general, even universal concerns.

Finally, my spiritual life also had to be examined because when I was much younger my relationship with God was very troubled. Talks with vicars as well as psychical research and readings in theology have all been helpful in changing my attitude to God. In subtle ways He has also revealed himself to me especially at very critical moments in my life. All of these things have helped to move me away from the empty, crass mentality I had had induced into me as a young man.

My healing therefore has had to progress on many levels but there is no doubt that my own episode had meaning in terms of my interior life and that examining the realm of meaning was vital, indeed indispensable, to recovery.

Peter interviewed by Sarah

Peter Chadwick suffered a psychotic episode in the summer of 1979 and has been well ever since. Since then he has put a lot of energy into the academic exploration of his illness and he feels that suffering psychosis has given him an insight into psychotic life. He says: '*It was with stress that I wrote some of these papers. But I thought if I don't do it, nobody else will*'. He was concerned with looking at the sufferer in as positive way as possible – something he felt was neglected by academic literature. He felt researchers were putting patients down in order to feed their own egos. Before the illness he was '*always working things out. I had to have a theory to live by, I couldn't just live*', but after the episode his attitude greatly changed.

He says that before he was put on a course of medication he was: '*hit by every small ripple in life*' Now he feels he is stronger and more able to cope with what life throws at him. The '*empty feeling of self*' that he had was all wiped away by medication. Peter is a '*card carrying believer*' in medication. He achieved his 'eureka' moment after prescription, whereas, he points out, '*They* [therapists] *would have you in therapy for years to solve the problem.*'

He had a double problem; he suffered from Tourette's syndrome and psychosis. '*I didn't know what was wrong with me. Nobody seemed to know about Tourette's in those days.*' When he found out what the appropriate medication was, his urgent reaction was, *'Can I take this drug right now?'* With haloperidol, which is the drug that he was prescribed, he experiences a small hit after about 20 minutes. He was sitting alone on a bus when the drug first took effect. He says, *'The moment it hit in my brain, I said to myself "it's all over" ... It just seemed to correct something. It put things right.'*

He feels that it's easy to write just about recovery. He argues that it is more important that people relate their experiences of the illness to their own lives, which is something that is seldom if ever done. By looking at the thought patterns and feelings that led you into the illness and asking questions such as, *'Where did it all come from?'* and *'Why did it overwhelm you?'* he feels you can start to tackle the really difficult issues. He says, *'It's a matter of how much insight you've got. We know very little about insight itself. It's up to you as to whether or not you're prepared to go into it in that way. How could you be so wrong? I admit there's a humiliating side to losing your sanity.'* But ultimately he feels that without knowing how you got there, you won't fully get better.

Though Peter recognises that a lot of 'emotional agony' is involved in making sense of what happened, he feels that the medication helps with this. He claims that it helps to make you stronger and more able to deal with the emotional issues that tackling 'why you got ill?' throws up. He is scathing about what he calls 'idealistic' psychoanalysts who say that you need to come off medication completely in order to have therapy. He points out that they are talking about something of which they have no experience – like a football manager who has never played football in his life.

His experience of psychosis left him with the feeling that he should suffer. He felt that he had to pay for his misspent life and his delusional beliefs were basically modelled on the people who had persecuted him in the past.

As well as suffering with Tourette's syndrome, Peter was a transvestite when he was younger. This was something that throughout his life he feels he has been stigmatised for more than his psychosis. Persecution for this feminine quality and not being sure he validly existed, which was a feeling he believes his mother instilled in him, stuck with him to the extent that it played out in his delusions. The delusions ultimately led to him throwing himself under a bus in 1979. He survived the collision, but his right hand was crushed and the right side of his torso and head scratched. He wrote to the bus driver to thank him for saving his life. This dramatic culmination of his illness meant that he had treatment and was prescribed the drugs that he felt made such a monumental difference to his life.

However when he left he was discharged to a hostel but he went to live with his girlfriend Jill instead: a woman he met in the day hospital, who is now his wife. He was lucky in this respect as he says that, '*Poor accommodation and financial difficulties and no one to properly talk to, are barriers to recovery.*'

It was important for him to mix with people who 'mirrored back' his own qualities. He adds, '*Meeting your wife is an absolutely amazing advantage*'. He and Jill 'clicked' really well, they could talk to each other about anything.

His psychosis also brought with it a faith in God. He says, '*It planted a seed in me of spiritual awareness.*' He feels that scientific enquiry had dulled his spirituality. With psychosis, '*You feel as though God and Satan are there with you as if behind a thin membrane. It changed me*'. Now he has no doubt that God exists, though he doesn't subscribe to organised religion. God has given meaning to his life, which he feels scientific training took away from him.

He does not see his psychotic episode as all bad. It changed him from a purely scientific mentality to one that he feels is fuller and better. After his episode he says he changed everything in his life, apart from his sex and his bank. He says, '*Before the illness I wasn't really myself*'. He doesn't think that many people can turn a psychotic experience around in this way, and estimates only 5–8% of people become better after psychosis than they were before.

He is reticent about calling himself a recovery hero. He says, '*At my age you don't usually have any heroes … not even yourself. I'm a person who's done well to get back into life.*' Peter feels he has lived a diverse and interesting life. He says, '*I've lived on my passions. I've lived a life where I've ridden on my feelings, particularly since my psychosis.*'

An appraisal of Peter by Jerome

Peter was born in Manchester in 1946, one of two sons, though his brother was 27 years older than him. His father died when he was only seven, leaving him to be brought up by his mother with whom he had a very complex relationship. After completing his education at North Manchester Grammar, he did a BSc in Geology at University College of Wales, Aberystwyth. He then did an MSc in Structural Geology at Imperial College and finally his PhD at the University of Liverpool. His geology research led to two papers in *Nature*, the most prestigious scientific journal in the world. A bright career in Geology must have beckoned and yet he decided to switch specialisms, and did a second undergraduate degree in Psychology at Bristol University, graduating with a first class honours in 1975. In the years that followed, he obtained a second PhD at the University of London in 1989 and a DSc in 2007 from Bristol University, both in psychology.

Peter's psychotic breakdown in 1979 and his subsequent treatment led to a lifelong interest in psychosis. Many of his books and articles combine insights obtained through his own personal experience of illness, along with his scholarly grasp of psychology, philosophy and literature in general. Unlike most researchers, virtually all his publications are single authorships, making his total of over 100 papers and books even more impressive.

Peter described his own recovery thus:

'[It] ... *has required chemotherapy (haloperidol), painful insight, the clarification of what is internal and what is external, or so-called reality testing, and non-possessive love from my close friends and from my wife – who acted as equals not superiors. It also required, however, a low expressed emotion home environment with my wife, forgiveness and real spiritual development, gradual re-employment, positive life enhancing coincidences, increased knowledge about psychosis and neurosis, a supportive GP and plenty of opportunity to talk about the crisis, to become fluent in it, to see even the comedy in it and the chance to relate it to my life as a whole...*' (Chadwick, 1993).

Peter was writing about the concept of recovery long before the topic had become as important as it is now. His main influences in the field have been as a teacher and lecturer, and as a writer. He has held a range of teaching posts both prior to and following his psychotic breakdown. He has written several books on psychosis (Chadwick, 1992, 1995, 1997, 2001 & 2009).

Peter's writings have to my mind been some of the most moving and inspirational in the field of mental health. Like Laing (1970), he has shown us how psychosis can also uplift. He is a true recovery hero.

Conclusion

Peter's recovery was aided by a number of factors; his creativity, his spirituality, an accepting loving relationship and even a small dose of neuroleptic medication. He found that attitudes were more stigmatising towards his previous experiences of transvestism, than towards his psychosis. He estimates that for between 5–8% of sufferers, psychosis can be a positive experience as it was for him. His writings have been hugely influential and he was one of the four recovery heroes who inspired Premila Trivedi.

References

Berrios G (1991) Delusions as wrong beliefs: a conceptual history. *British Journal of Psychiatry* **159** (14) 16–3.

Chadwick P (1992) *Borderline: A psychological study of paranoia and delusional thinking*. London: Routledge.

Chadwick P (1993) The stepladder to the impossible: a first hand phenomenological account of a schizoaffective psychotic crisis. *Journal of Mental Health* **2** 239–250.

Chadwick P (1995) *Understanding Paranoia: What causes it, how it feels and what to do about it?* London: Thorsons.

Chadwick P (1997) *Schizophrenia – The Positive Perspective: In search of dignity for schizophrenic people*. London: Routledge.

Chadwick P (2001) *Personality as Art: Artistic approaches in psychology*. Ross-on-Wye: PCCS Books.

Chadwick P (2009) *Schizophrenia – The Positive Perspective: Explorations at the outer reaches of human experience*. Second edition. London: Routledge.

Laing RD (1970) *The Divided Self*. London: Pelican.

Chapter 7

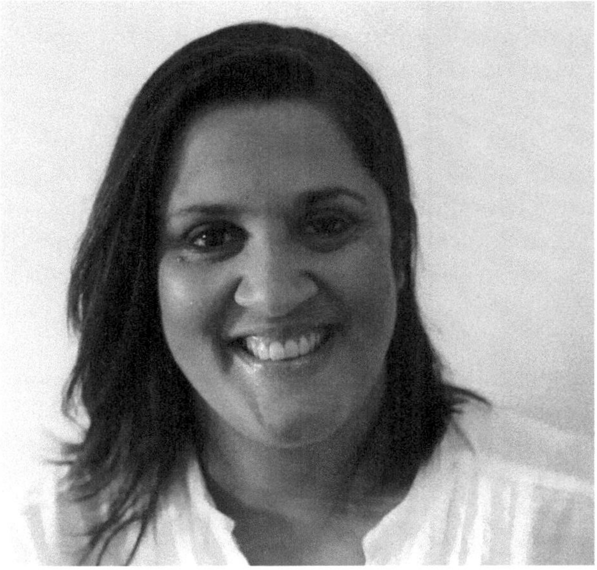

Dolly Sen

Summary

Dolly was brought up in almost Dickensian conditions and she developed a psychosis in her teenage years. Her recovery was a slow process and one which didn't start until she was in her 30s. Since then her progress has been remarkable. She went to university and obtained a first class honours degree and she now works in the country's first ever Recovery Education Centre as a peer trainer.

Dolly in her own words

Dolly Sen was born in 1970 in London and was the oldest of five children. She is from a mixed heritage; her father is Indian and her mother is Scots-Irish. Her childhood was not a happy one with physical, emotional, mental, sexual abuse, racism, poverty, neglect and bullying. Despite this, she excelled academically and had very close bonds with her siblings.

When Dolly was 14 years old she had her first psychotic episode and had to drop out of school. She was under the care of child psychiatry and social services but felt that they exacerbated her problems by trying to force her back into the school system, without addressing either the volatile home situation or the psychosis.

Dolly attempted to work but was unable to as she was lost in a world of psychosis, self-harm and suicide attempts until her 30s. She has been in hospital four times in 2000, 2001, 2005 and 2006 and is currently diagnosed with bipolar affective disorder, but in the past she had been diagnosed with schizophrenia and psychotic depression.

Three things changed this darkness into light, and these were her decision to recover and take personal responsibility, her creativity, and a course of cognitive behaviour therapy in the Psychological Interventions Clinic for Outpatients with Psychosis Clinic (PICuP) at The Maudsley Hospital.

This enabled her to dream and to make up for three decades of painful sleep – now Dolly is an accomplished and published writer and her works include, *The World is Full of Laughter* (Sen, 2002) and *Am I Still Laughing?* (Sen, 2006).

Dolly's dreams keep coming and keep being lived. She is a writer, director, artist, film-maker, poet, performer, raconteur, playwright, mental health consultant, music-maker and public speaker. These include a succession of performance roles around Europe and at places like The Young Vic, Trafalgar Square and The Royal Festival Hall. She has undertaken a poetry tour and won a poetry award from Andrew Motion. She directed two plays and several films, appeared on TV, and she has presented at City Hall, London, and Oxford University. She has appeared on TV and radio over 20 times talking about mental health issues. This is quite staggering because in the past she was told she would never amount to anything but would end up in jail or Broadmoor. She believed this and was on her way there until she changed her belief into one of believing she could do anything she wanted to do. To Dolly, this proves that the mind is an amazing thing; it can drive you mad and inspire you in the same breath. Also it proves that you can do anything if you believe you can do it.

Dolly interviewed by Sarah

Dolly Sen spent years in a delusional state. She published her book *The World is Full of Laughter* in 2002 to much acclaim. Most recently she performed at Bonkersfest, a festival by and for the mentally ill. In the programme she calls herself a professional mad person. She tells me that since she's been creative professionally, she writes, talks and creates artwork around the subject of being ill, '*I just find I'm being paid for being mad,*' she laughs.

She describes how she first got ill: '*I was listening to the top 40 on the radio, when … the DJ's voice kind of disappeared and instead this kind of deep gravely male voice began talking to me and saying you know I'm watching you, I know what you want.*' She says, '*Those two sentences were the very first sentences of me hearing voices.*'

She experienced one long period of psychosis from that point. '*It was basically like that block of time was my 20s and a little bit of my late teenage years. I wasn't Dolly Sen, I was this thing taken over by psychosis. Paranoid and depressed and angry and negative … the only kind of light I had in those days was my writing … it stopped me going too into myself. But then again, having said that, when you're really ill you can't write.*'

She was very embarrassed about her illness and didn't talk to her family about it. Talking about her family in her first mental health memoir forced her family to talk about it. '*You know after that I felt really supported by my family,*' she says.

Once her illness was more public she had both positive and negative reactions to it. She used to have a neighbour who reported her to the Department for Social Security (DSS). The neighbour wrote threatening notes and Dolly even had faeces put through her letter box. That was the worst example, but usually reactions are less extreme. She also gets people saying, '*I'm going to make something of my life after reading your story*'.

While Dolly first saw a psychiatrist at 14 because the paranoia stopped her going to school, she didn't admit to hearing voices or having hallucinations, so she was just treated for depression and she didn't take her medication. She says it was only in her 20s when she '*just wanted help*' that she went to her GP and was transferred to the Mental Health Centre. It was only after six weeks of taking antidepressants and seeing a key worker that she admitted to seeing and hearing things and was put on antipsychotics.

She has been hospitalised several times. '*There were a lot of women who were really vulnerable because there were men that would pester them. I was big and crazy enough to tell them to F off.*' As a result she feels hospitalisation wasn't good for her recovery, '*Let me put it this way, they said: "Dolly are you hearing voices or do you think that people are coming to get you?" And I said no, even though I believed it. I just wanted to get out as quickly as possible.*' She was back in the hospital two weeks later.

Dolly was first in hospital for three months, then six weeks, then a month and finally three weeks. '*I don't plan to go back in, so I'm not going to say it's going to get better each time* [the length of her hospital stays].' She says, '*I've had a lot* [of antipsychotics] *because they weren't working. It was eight years until they found the right one. That's a lot of time to wait, actually.*'

She had to fight for non-drug therapies. In her 20s she asked eight different psychiatrists for cognitive behavioural therapy (CBT), and was told by all of them that it was only for people with depression and it couldn't help her. They said the same about psychotherapy. It was only when she had a 'good' psychiatrist that she got put on the waiting list for CBT at the clinic at the Maudsley hospital. She was on the waiting list a year.

She says, '*CBT was the first thing that made me see that my psychotic thinking was actually quite logical and it always followed the same pattern. What CBT does is to show how one thought affects another and affects another and then you end up in the midst of paranoia or kind of depression. What the service did was break down this thinking process but with alternatives.*'

She felt a lot of people outside the mental health service helped her recovery like her publisher, Jason Pegler, '*He was the first person to really truly believe, not just the fact that I could be a good writer. He believed that I could recover, nobody else had that belief about me, not even me.*' He persuaded her to write her life story for Chipmunka Press, which concerned her at first because her life had been so difficult. But once started, she finished the book in six weeks. '*That's how much it needed to get out.*' There is a note of laughter in her voice. '*It was a cathartic experience.*'

At the same time Dolly became one of the founding members of Creative Routes who organise the Bonkersfest, which started at the end of 2002. Their original membership of six is now around 500. She feels the artists she has met have helped her. '*I had social phobia for the longest time and I met a poet who kind of literally forced me onto the stage,*' she laughs, '*to do some of my poetry reading*'. They helped by giving her confidence. For her, the artists she has met have been the biggest influence on her, as unlike mental health professionals, she says, '*They do see my heart and they do see I'm a human being and that I've got good things inside me. They don't see something that's broken, they see someone who can make poetry and music and write. I call them my angels actually.*'

She says that with some mental health professionals, '*It's like you're being served at Woolworths. Sometimes what you just need is a hug from these people.*' She had a more positive relationship with the woman who gave her CBT, '*That was probably one of the first times in the system where I felt this person had hope for me.*' This female professional said Dolly simply needed strategies to improve her quality of life and in order to get her symptoms under control.

For her, being well is having control of her life and control over her symptoms, '*Wellness is being able to laugh about yourself, because I think you really need that. Just to see that my dreams, they're not going to stay in my head, they're going to come true.*'

An appraisal of Dolly Sen by Jerome

Shortly after I moved from the Norwood Team to work in the Streatham Service in South London, I began to hear about Dolly Sen. Colleagues would tell me in almost reverential tones how '*she had written a book*.' The opportunity to meet Dolly came when I invited her to give a talk at our local Recovery Group (Morgan & Carson, 2008). She spoke to a group of our service users and answered a whole range of questions from how she coped with suicidal thoughts, to the importance of having dreams for your life. '*Have big dreams, take small steps*', she advised. She came back a couple of years later to give a second presentation on doing her video and film degree, for which she was awarded a first class honours degree. Our service users were hugely inspired by her presence and personal witness.

The story of Dolly's life and illness as revealed in her two books is a remarkable account of recovery, not just from mental illness, but extreme social adversity. Her story is an example of what the journalist India Knight (2008) has referred to as Mislit (Misery Literature), which I note Waterstones places in a section called, 'Painful Lives'. Her life was as painful a story as I had ever heard in my years as a clinical psychologist.

This woman happened to be a service user in the new community mental health team I was working in, and was our own local recovery hero. Another service user, Michelle McNary (see Chapter 10) has made a film about recovery, which features Dolly and three other local service users. In the booklet that accompanies the film (Carson *et al*, 2008) Dolly describes what helped her recover:

'In the fabric of hell that enclosed me like a straitjacket, there was an infinitesimal tear, a hole which unraveled my hell, thread by thread, until the constraints became more whole than limitation ... Recovery is a letter of hopes, dreams, songs, peace, hurt, chaos, transcendence, night and light. Recovery is to be able to dream and live those dreams. To shine my brightest and live my fullest. To seize the day without the weight of the past. To lose any negativity in my life. To find the Dollyness of Dolly,' (Sen, 2008).

The four key elements of recovery according to Andresen *et al* (2003) are having hope, finding meaning in life, developing a sense of identity separate from an illness and taking personal responsibility for your life. These are complex processes. To my mind, Dolly epitomises all four summed up in her wonderful phrase, '*To find the Dollyness of Dolly*'. Patricia Deegan also reminds us that the most important goal is '*to become the unique, awesome, never to be repeated human being that we are called to be,*' (Deegan, 1996). The challenge for all of us is to help our service users value their own uniqueness and help them move towards their own personal dreams and goals. Dolly Sen is a remarkable woman. To my mind, she is a true recovery hero.

Conclusion

Dolly Sen's progress towards recovery did not start until she was 30. Since then she has written several books on her own story and experiences, and she has also appeared in several films about psychosis. She is now a peer trainer in the Recovery Education Centre, currently located in the grounds of Springfield Hospital.

For more information about Dolly, check out her website: http://www.dollysen.com.

References

Andresen R, Caputi P & Oades L (2003) The experience of recovery from schizophrenia: towards an empirically validated stage model. *Australian and New Zealand Journal of Psychiatry* **37** 586–594.

Carson J, Holloway F, Wolfson P & McNary M (Eds) (2008) *Recovery Journeys: Stories of coping with mental health problems*. London: South London and Maudsley NHS Foundation Trust.

Deegan P (1996) Recovery as a journey of the heart. *Psychiatric Rehabilitation Journal* **11** 11–19.

Knight I (2008) Our taste for all this misery lit makes ugly reading. *The Sunday Times*. November 23rd.

Morgan S & Carson J (2008) The Recovery Group: a service user and professional perspective. *Groupwork* **19** (1) 26–39.

Sen D (2002) *The World is Full of Laughter*. Brentwood: Chipmunka Press.

Sen D (2006) *Am I Still Laughing?* Brentwood: Chipmunka Press.

Sen D (2008) *Dolly's Story*. In: J Carson, F Holloway, P Wolfson & M McNary (Eds) (2008) *Recovery Journeys: Stories of coping with mental health problems*. London: South London and Maudsley NHS Foundation Trust.

Chapter 8

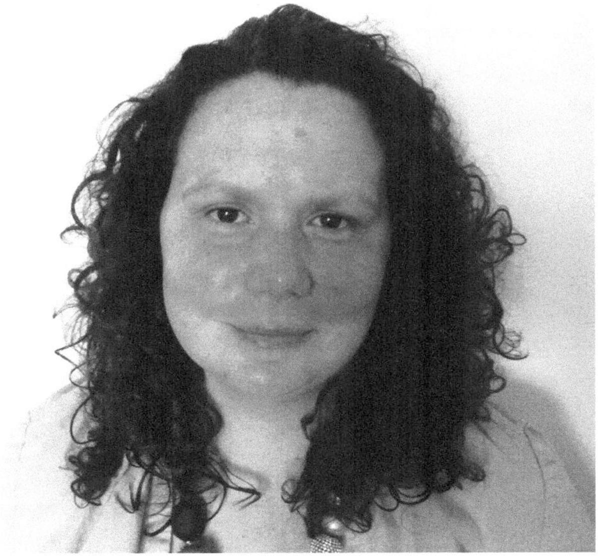

Emma Harding

Summary

Emma Harding had a psychotic breakdown during her undergraduate degree, but she eventually returned to complete her studies. Rachel Perkins appointed her to a job as part of her own mission to enable service users to access jobs in mental health services. Emma's promotional work on service user perspectives led to her being asked to apply for a clinical psychology training place. Now she is successfully employed as a clinical psychologist in the health service and she is in an ideal position to help bring about the transition in mental health services that is so sorely needed, if services are to become truly transformative.

Emma in her own words

I struggle to think of myself as a hero, but am far too self-indulgent to turn down the opportunity to sit alongside the other far more deserving individuals included in this book.

I became unwell as a teenager when I was studying for an undergraduate degree in social psychology, although the decline into insanity started some time before, as it became apparent in hindsight. I think I chose to study psychology to see if I was normal as well, because I found people tended to like to tell me their 'stuff'. (I have since concluded that there are so few 'normal' people, and in fact they are really the 'weird' ones). I also remember pondering as a child whether the brain or the heart was the most crucial human organ, and was quite pleased with myself when I decided the former commanded more authority over life. However, had I decided the heart was more important I don't think I would have chosen to be a physician – I find blood and related fluids far more stomach-turning than the most esoteric delusional thinking.

I chose to work in mental health services for many reasons; the admirable ones being to make a difference and help people, the more self-serving relating to my experience being hugely meaningful and significant, to me anyway. I wanted, in some way, to dwell on it and make it useful – to mark it in some way. It is (now) quite amusing to me to think that I thought I was God (having swallowed the guilt) – and I should probably spend more time trying to uncover why my psyche chose that particular way to preserve itself. Effectively, some unconscious element put my fragile, emergent self under a protective shell and went all out to distract potentially harmful influences from it by putting on a gaudy, larger than life 'show' of being a deity. Humour, selective attention and an acquired thick skin tend to get me through the 'shame attack' of embarrassing memories that periodically make me squirm.

'Recovery' is not exactly easy, and many people struggle to distance themselves from distress. In many ways I have been lucky, benefiting from a loving family and partner, excellent education, freedom from most forms of socio-economic difficulty and, forgive the pun, the luck of the Gods. Although I have also had some extreme experiences of psychosis, these factors have protected me from getting permanently lost in them. Having, as one fellow 'inmate' put it: *'stared into the void'* and made it back, I remain eager to share my interpretation of madness and indulge my curiosity in others by involving myself as far as possible in developing stories or explanations of people's mental crises, in turn enriching my understanding of this fundamentally human condition.

People often say that it must be frightening to learn about mental illness when you have it yourself, I would disagree – although lots of us just don't want any further information about it, thank you very much. I worked in a programme pioneered by the amazing Rachel Perkins, also a contributor to this book, which sought to support people with mental health problems to work in NHS mental health services, and I owe a lot to Rachel for starting and propelling my career. I was often asked about stigma from colleagues who find themselves working alongside members of staff who are mad. I find these days I am more bothered by the few clients I work with who assume that as a member of staff, I obviously haven't heard voices or felt suicidal or soul-rending metaphysical isolation. Some instead have intimated that individual service providers should absorb all criticism and blame. I choose not to volunteer information about my mental health problems to users of my team's services – either for sympathy or to suggest I might know what they are going through, but no service provider I know is immune or indifferent to pain.

Rachel Perkins has been a leading light in making it unremarkable for us 'nutters' to be working in mental health services from an organisational point of view. By sharing my story, I get to congratulate myself again on making it out alive, but it also might leave mental distress seeming just that little bit less unusual. Hopefully the proliferation of accounts of psychosis will soon be so common they become boring, but at the time of writing, the exercise is still a little brave for a psychologist ('brave' being a word I consider substituting 'stupid' in this context). Eventually (hopefully) madness will be accepted, expected and respected and people living with it won't stigmatise themselves, assume they are separate from 'normal' people or that they are alone. By contributing to this book I hope to add my voice to the growing numbers of those who want to point out what a 'normal' experience madness is.

I haven't said so much about my background in this account, but I have wanted to explain myself and my involvement in this book more generally. To summarise my position, I am unashamedly going to steal someone else's quotation. As George Mallory is reputed to have said about climbing Everest, I fight my own and others' mental illness and stigma '*because it is there*' (Holzel & Salked, 2000). Unlike Everest, it shouldn't be.

Emma interviewed by Sophie

Her descent into psychosis took clinical psychologist Emma Harding by total surprise. Having always considered herself independent, down to earth and not especially unusual or 'random' in her own words, she was overtaken in the first year of university by a series of strange experiences and what was finally diagnosed as schizophrenia.

She first noticed that something was untoward when she was bawling her eyes out in the car on the way from home in Cambridge to university in Canterbury, aged 18. At university she immediately wanted people to like her and to fit in, yet she found herself completely overwhelmed by the plethora of new people. Back at home she had rebelled and got in with a very different crowd to the sort she was now meeting at university, which she found confusing. What's more, all the challenges presented by having to look after herself for the first time, like doing her own laundry and cooking added to the difficulty.

'I really wanted people to like me but I felt like I wasn't ever going to be one of them. I started dissecting conversations and second guessing other people and finding evidence for them not liking me. So I'd start to stay in lots and listen to music on my own. That's when I started hearing voices – I couldn't at that stage quite hear what they were saying but they definitely sounded quite frightening,' she said.

Emma started trying to self-diagnose by reading up on what might be wrong. She resorted to the university's phone line counselling service but found it of no help. Before long she was much worse and with work pressure on top of everything else that was bothering her – essays were becoming more and more difficult – she decided that it would be better for everyone concerned if she killed herself. She took an overdose of Prozac and was immobilised on her own in her room for three whole days. That was in March of her first year, but somehow she found the strength to go back to college and take exams a few months later in May. When Emma went home for the summer, the voices got more real, and in some cases, more bizarre. She started, for instance, to think that she alone could control lamp posts.

Everything came to a head when Emma had an 'epiphany' in which she experienced a total revelation about herself and her place in the world. *'One day everything suddenly revealed itself to me. I believed wholeheartedly for three months that I was God. I didn't tell people because I thought everyone knew already through a sort of unconscious 'matrix' system. I believed everything had a life force, and drew eyes on the hoover as it obviously needed them,'* she said. Watching the news became terrifying as Emma started to believe she was spiritually responsible for many of the harrowing things that were happening around the world, such as an earthquake in Japan.

One salvation in this torment proved to be the church. Emma went to see the clergy in her local church and met a vicar who gave her an absolution. The vicar was '*very calming and lovely*' in Emma's words and gave her a crucifix on a necklace that she came to treasure. At this point, Emma was still not diagnosed with schizophrenia. When her father took her to see the family GP, they were told that Emma herself would need to say that she had a problem for there to be any specialist investigation. Finally, that diagnosis came towards the end of 1994, when the psychiatrist visited Emma in her house and saw her worsening condition.

Remarkably, despite being in hospital for about two months, Emma managed to go back to college and finish her psychology degree. The university was initially not keen to have her back, because they were worried about her condition. However, Emma had regained a lot of confidence while in hospital. She had also, at day hospital, received help with study skills, including advice and encouragement on how to tackle exams. The psychiatrist felt she would be better off deferring, but Emma preferred to push on, and finished her degree in 1997 – just two years after coming out of hospital.

After experiencing such profound experiences so young, Emma wanted to do something personally important with her life. She dismissed the idea of becoming a clinical psychologist because lecturers cautioned that it would be impossible to get into. Instead, she followed up on an article her father read about people with mental health problems being employed to help others with mental health conditions within mental health services.

She began work as a mental health support worker in Tooting, South London, having been interviewed by Dr Rachel Perkins. She then moved on to work for Rachel's team supporting other employees. During those 18 months, she began public speaking, getting involved in training programmes and thinking about service user empowerment issues in general. Those skills became very useful shortly after, when she began to volunteer for Rethink. She began engaging with more and more public speaking, including TV and radio appearances, for which she developed a real passion.

One pivotal day, Emma was giving training when she happened to meet a trainee clinical psychologist who asked her to get involved in advising universities on how service users and trainers can become more involved in providing care. Initially unsure about taking part, on the advice of her partner, she took up the opportunity. That decision turned out to be a very important one when one day, at one of the meetings, she met a clinical psychologist who encouraged her to apply for clinical psychology training herself. The psychologist believed it would be refreshing to train more psychologists with more than a textbook understanding of mental health problems. It also happened to be the time of year when applications were due. In a supreme turn around, Emma now trained to be a clinical psychologist and, after three years of training, qualified in 2008.

Since qualifying, Emma has been working at the South London and Maudsley NHS Trust. For anyone who chooses to Google her, there is ample evidence on the internet of her personal experiences of psychosis. However Emma doesn't want to make her past too high profile for fear of being labelled the 'schizophrenic who is also a professional' and hence potentially denting her professional profile. She prefers to be known as a 'professional who happens to have experienced mental health problems'. On the other hand, Emma is wary of hiding her mental health issues from service users, since she does not want to send out the wrong message about promoting honesty and openness about mental health problems.

Emma's life has transformed once more in the last few months with the birth of her first child. When she's ready to go back to work, no doubt she will enjoy her line of work as much as ever, informed as it is by her own experiences. '*Sometimes it really helps to have a sense that however nonsensical someone's beliefs sound, if you listen enough, they actually do always make sense. Also if someone is being particularly resistant or rude, I would want to work hard to see the situation from their perspective to help develop more patience. Having experienced the receiving end of care, I imagine myself in their shoes, even if that means sometimes I'm too much on the side of the patient rather than the service, as someone has to be!*' she comments.

An appraisal of Emma by Jerome

I first met Emma Harding in a first class departure lounge at Heathrow Airport. We were both travelling out to Portugal to speak at a small seminar for a group of drug reps. Emma was going along with a Rethink worker to provide a service user perspective. I performed so poorly during my own presentation that I was dropped off the speaker's rota and was never invited back. Before going back to London, I was able to listen to Emma's presentation. Not for the first time I was transfixed by the articulacy and persuasiveness with which a service user presenter spoke about their experiences of psychosis and contact with mental health services. Emma told the drug reps about her breakdown, hospitalisation and subsequent on-going recovery (see accounts which she has written, Harding, 2009; Harding, 2011). I could never have imagined, as I sat there that day, that a decade or so later she would be one of my professional clinical psychology colleagues at the Maudsley.

There are of course clear parallels with Emma's story and that of Rufus May (see Chapter 16), but there are obvious contrasts in how they present themselves. As Emma says in her interview, she does not want to be known as 'the schizophrenic who is also a professional' but as a 'professional who happens to have experienced mental health problems'. This contrasts with the headlines generated by Rufus, '*The mad doctor: the extraordinary story of Dr Rufus May, the former psychiatric patient*' (The Independent, 2007).

When Emma first came to work at the Maudsley I arranged to take her out for lunch. I had hoped to try and persuade her to come along and speak about her experiences at one of our recovery groups. She did not feel established or secure enough in her new role to be able to say yes at that point. Some months later when I asked her to contribute to our new book, *Psychosis Stories of Recovery and Hope* (2011), she was again a little reticent. However, I pointed out to her that she had just had a paper published in that month's Clinical Psychology Forum talking about her experiences as a service user. I said, '*Emma every psychologist in the country knows about you now!*' Luckily, I won the day and the book, as like this book it is the richer for having her contribution and reflections.

Emma talks openly about the difficulties of 'coming out' about a history of mental health problems. Not only might this create problems with professional colleagues, but some service users might feel uncomfortable working with a professional who has similar problems to them. The clinical service is however enriched by having someone like Emma in it who has a desire to help individuals understand their psychotic experiences. I for one look forward to reading more of her work in the future as I am convinced that she will continue to make outstanding contributions to our understanding of psychosis.

Conclusion

Mental health professionals working with people with psychosis are at a profound disadvantage: most of us have no idea what it is like to hear voices or to suffer with extreme delusional beliefs. Emma had a psychotic breakdown while an undergraduate. She could not have envisaged then that her recovery would lead to her training later in life as a clinical psychologist. She is thus in an ideal position to help sufferers with psychosis having gone through similar experiences herself. Already through her writing she has raised awareness of the barriers that many sufferers face in their recovery. She has also shown how meeting with key individuals in her own recovery journey has helped her get to where she is today. I believe we are still to see the best from Emma Harding. However, the hardest attitudes to changing services to become more recovery focused may be in changing the attitudes of the professionals who work within them.

References

Harding E (2009) Recovery – adventures in being. In: R Chandler & M Hayward (Eds) *Voicing Psychotic Experiences: A reconsideration of recovery and diversity*. Brighton: Pavilion Publishing.

Harding E (2011) A psychologist's progress. In: H Cordle, J Fradgley, J Carson, Holloway F & Richards P (Eds) *Psychosis Stories of Recovery and Hope*. London: Quay Books.

Holzel T & Salked A (2000) *The Mystery of Mallory and Irvine*. Seattle: The Mountaineers.

May R (2007) The Mad Doctor: the extraordinary story of Dr Rufus May, the former psychiatric patient. The *Independent* March 18th.

Chapter 9

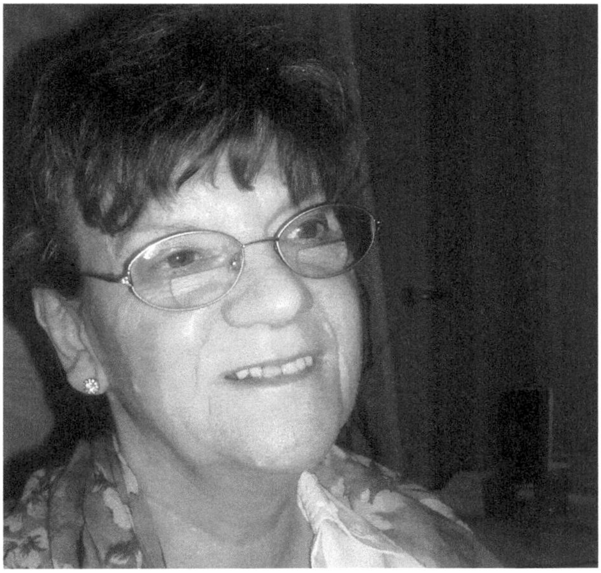

Margaret Muir

Summary

Margaret Muir has been involved in recovery work for the last four years. She has claimed that all service users are recovery heroes and in this she echoes the views of the American clinical psychologist, Dr Patricia Deegan. She describes her own difficult upbringing and the tragic death of her sister when she was just a child herself. She has developed interests in photography and in delivering a gratitude intervention to other service users.

Margaret in her own words

I was born in 1943 during World War II and I was the eldest of two daughters. On Christmas Eve 1948, my little sister Pauline was born. The following spring we moved from Belgravia to St Margarets near Richmond. We had an idyllic life until November 1952, when after a very short illness, Pauline tragically died. I remember that time vividly even to this day. On Christmas Day we packed our bags and went to stay with my aunt and uncle and two cousins. I attended my cousin's school and hated every minute. The school was a large four or five storey dismal grey Victorian building, much different from my bungalow school back home, and I missed my friends. When we came home the following May, my mother went out to work full time and I became a very lonely 'latch key' kid. I started having nightmares, sleep walking and felt the world wasn't real and neither were the people in it. Nobody talked to me about Pauline and I could not talk to my parents. As young as I was, I could see the pain etched on their faces, their grief was beyond imagination. My grief stayed locked away inside me for many years to come. I miss my little sister to this day and often think of what could have been.

I married young and gave birth to three beautiful daughters and I enjoyed being a mother. I cannot bring myself to write much about my marriage only to say that he (my now ex-husband) was violent and we all went through hell. I think that explains enough. After 17 years of marriage I asked him to leave, and much to our surprise he did.

Two years later my kind and gentle father died. It was a great shock to me as he looked too young to die, he was only 68. My Dad's death was a tremendous loss and I shed many tears. This was another bereavement that I experienced but as my children were still at home, I had a lot of support from them.

In September 1995, I started to feel suicidal. In January 1996, my mother died, and I had spent three weeks in hospital by her bedside. While she was dying and after her death, I became extremely unwell. I had been depressed for about eight years before, but this time it was a rapid descent into some kind of madness. I had a few hallucinations which paralysed me with fear. It was 'not me in my head', I felt suicidal, had nightmares (which lasted five years) and severe depression. I spent a lot of time in bed over the next four years and went out under cover of darkness to do my food shopping. I was in deep agonising despair and I had lost my dreams.

After three years I was referred to see a psychiatrist. Two years on, I was admitted into hospital three times in one year. When I was in there, I had a few hallucinations. I think they were due to a new medication, which was Venlafaxine. After two weeks I was diagnosed with depersonalisation disorder with severe depression. The psychiatrist will never know how relieved I was, as this explained so many of my symptoms including the 'not me in my head', which was the loss of personal identity. My symptoms were caused by all the traumatic events that happened over many years.

Losing a loved one is agony in the extreme. The loss of my sister and mother made me particularly ill. In later years these experiences gave me more insight into the grief of others. I have discovered that 'grief takes as long as it takes'.

I am very fortunate and thankful for all the things I have in my life. I now focus on what I have in life and not what's missing. I have three lovely daughters, six beautiful grandchildren and an adorable great grandson.

I believe all who suffer the pain and anguish of mental illness are heroes. Anyone who has survived weeks, months or even years in mental institutions are heroes. Anyone who has spent years dragging themselves out of the abyss is a hero. Some of us lose family and friends and are not even treated as human beings. These people are the unsung heroes.

Margaret interviewed by Hannah Cordle

After two years in the recovery movement, Margaret Muir is in a unique position. When we meet, she had just been named 'Woman of the Year' at the first Recovery Awards held by the South West Sector Community Mental Health Team. Designed to recognise and reward outstanding personal achievement in the area of recovery, the award confirms that Margaret is a true recovery hero. She is surprised and humbled that her efforts have been recognised, despite obviously having worked hard for the honour. '*I just enjoy doing it!*' she says. '*It keeps me busy and I believe in the work, but I didn't know it was being recognised. But as far as I'm concerned there are lots of people here doing excellent work, perhaps not in the same way.*'

Margaret came to the recovery movement after experiencing what she describes as nearly a lifetime of severe depression and also a diagnosis of depersonalisation disorder given to her nine years ago. The illness has at times made her feel suicidal, and she experienced depression, loss of identity and nightmares. After several months of working with her consultant clinical psychologist, Margaret began to attend the recovery group which is run at the Streatham team base. It was here she realised that her personal recovery had reached a plateau and that a different approach was needed for her to progress.

'I was just stuck and I had to be given the tools to work with,' she says. *'I realised that you can take the horse to water but you can't make it drink. That's when I started to think, "Well, I'm involved, I'm the only one who can really do the work, I need the tools to recover, but it needs me to do the work".'*

Despite knowing that recovery is a new thing in mental health, Margaret began to get more engaged with the work and started to see results. Like several other members of the recovery group, she made a personal presentation on recovery, Lessons from the University of Life, which led to her involvement in a variety of pioneering projects run at the Streatham team base.

Last year she took part in a pilot study on thankfulness where service users were asked to record three reasons to be thankful each day. Margaret admits that at first she did not think she would be able to do this, but with her characteristic determination, she was the only person to complete the project and eventually co-facilitated some workshops. *'I think it helped other people, I did get some thank you cards and one of them said I'd helped her and she's thankful for things she's never ever been thankful for before,'* (Carson *et al*, 2010a; 2010b).

The project also helped Margaret to appreciate many of the things in life – large and small – that she had forgotten about during her illness. *'I'm thankful for everything, thankful for the sunrise, sunset, moon, stars, even the foxes outside my French windows even though they're a pain in the neck!'* she laughs. *'It made me think about what I used to enjoy, what I got out of life. I couldn't see but that's all come back.'* Indulging her love of classical music and days out to her favourite places such as Richmond and Horsham are also ways that Margaret has found pleasure in life again.

Another sign of recovery for Margaret is that as a self-confessed dreamer, she is allowing herself to dream once again after years of *'seeing nothing'*. *'It's nice to have dreams such as a house in the country,'* she says. *'That's about hope as well, and my children to have the things that I'd like them to have, dreams for them and their family.'* She worked towards capturing her dreams in photographs through the Photographing Hope project, which was led by another service user. This involved service users taking a series of digital photographs on the theme of hope, which are exhibited at the Streatham team base. At the first workshop, Margaret encouraged her colleagues with a quote from Malcolm Forbes that '*When you cease to dream, you cease to live*' (Winans, 1990).

Margaret explains how pushing herself to complete these projects has helped her confidence grow and reduce her depression. '*Trying to do the things you're supposed to do – it took me a long time to learn this – is better than letting your emotions get the better of you and going into that stage of inertia,*' she says. '*Because it's better to push yourself, it's easier than to go into that state and mode of thinking.*'

'*With depression you can't do anything, nothing. And all the time you want to and it's like an anxiety because you want to do these things but you can't. But I'm saying it's better to do them, I felt more anxious not doing it.*'

Now recovery has taken on a new meaning for Margaret, who like many service users, at first considered the term to be misleading. '*The word recovery didn't sit well with me and to my mind at the time it meant cure,*' she explains. '*It suddenly hits you that it doesn't mean cure, but it means to basically cope with your symptoms. I was relieved when I heard this because I thought the expectation was that in a very short space of time I wouldn't have any symptoms of my illness ever again. I felt pressurised to get well completely.*' Now her definition of recovery is '*peace in my head, hope for the future, thankfulness that I am alive and laughing, which is really important*'.

She has also learned not to mix with people that bring her down or make her feel more anxious. She advises that '*there is no blueprint for recovery, everybody's recovery is unique, so go by what your heart tells you and if you don't understand, ask, which I made the mistake of not doing.*'

To someone entering mental health services, Margaret would hope to offer hope and inspiration. '*I'd say anything's possible although they might not feel it, and not to rush and not to feel pressurised into getting better too quickly, one step up the ladder but they are not failing if they fall. And to keep trying and don't give up, there is no shame in making mistakes, we learn by them, it's easier if you try than not.*' And from the Recovery Awards 'Woman of the Year', this is surely advice worth taking.

An appraisal of Margaret by Jerome

It was while we were having a meal to celebrate the end of two gratitude workshops when Margaret made her memorable comment. I had just persuaded Matt to agree to be the fourth recovery hero in our series, when Margaret commented from across the room, '*We're all recovery heroes!*'. She was of course correct.

In saying this, Margaret was echoing the views of Patricia Deegan. In helping students work more compassionately with service users, she commented: '*... I ask students to suspend their perception of people as chronic mental patients and to try and see the individual as a hero ... could you have survived what this individual has survived?*' (Deegan, 1996)

Margaret has been the mainstay of our local recovery group (Morgan & Carson, 2009). Since the group started in November 2007, she has missed only one session. She also told her own story in a presentation entitled, Lessons from the University of Life. In this talk, she divided her life into thirds; her childhood upbringing, her married life and her life since she separated from her husband. She brought along family photographs to illustrate each phase and used poetry and music to capture some of the feelings of each stage. She chose a number of brief statements to capture the meaning of each period. In her own piece in this chapter she states evocatively, '*Grief takes as long as it takes*'. Losing her sister at an early age no doubt led to this wisdom. Along with Gordon and Matt, Margaret helped me run a workshop at the Lambeth Recover Me conference. She also spoke at our World Mental Health day event. Together we ran two gratitude workshops for nine service users, based on the work of Professor Robert Emmons (2007). Given all of the above, Margaret was a natural choice for our Woman of the Year award at our first Recovery Group Oscars.

Since then, Margaret joined Matthew Ward and Elizabeth Wakely to present the work of the local recovery group at the 2010 European Groupwork Symposium in York, where Professor Johnson commented on Margaret's '*beautiful photography*' (Johnson, 2010). For someone whose education had been in the '*university of life*' this was a further step in Margaret's own recovery journey.

Conclusion

As so many have already said, recovery is hard work. This has certainly been the case for Margaret, who has not had the easiest of lives. The loss of her sister Pauline in childhood was a tragic loss for both her parents and herself. An unhappy and violent marriage was a further setback. Following the death of her mother, she went on to have further mental health problems with a number of hospital admissions. For the last four years she has been on a recovery journey and her inspiration has been a great encouragement to others. Her wisdom, '*Grief takes as long as it takes*', reminds us we cannot put a fixed time on bereavement. Similarly, she is surely right that anyone battling with a major mental disorder is a recovery hero.

References

Carson J, Muir Margaret M, Clark S, Wakely E & Chander A (2010a) Piloting a gratitude intervention in a community mental health team. *Groupwork* **20** (3) 73–87.

Carson J, Chander A, Muir M, Wakely E & Clark S (2010b) Silent gratitude isn't much use to anyone: piloting a gratitude intervention in a community mental health team. *Clinical Psychology Forum* **212** 27–31.

Deegan P (1996) Recovery as a journey of the heart. *Psychiatric Rehabilitation Journal* **19** (3) 91–97.

Emmons R (2007) *Thanks: How the new science of gratitude can make you happier*. New York: Houghton-Mifflin.

Johnson P (2010) Groupwork and wellbeing: 2010 European Groupwork Symposium, a personal account. *Groupwork* **20** (3) 115–119.

Morgan S & Carson J (2009) The Recovery group: a service user and professional perspective. *Groupwork* **19** (1) 26–39.

Winans C (1990) *Malcolm Forbes: The man who had everything*. New York: St Martin's Press.

Chapter 10

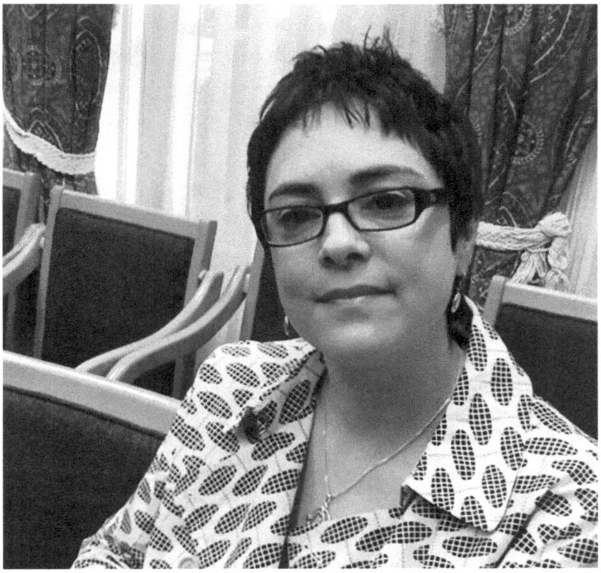

Michelle McNary

Summary

Michelle McNary spent over two years making the *Recovery* film. She persuaded two senior trust staff to commission the making of a film about recovery featuring only service users. The film was funded by the Charitable Trustees of the South London and Maudsley NHS Trust. Since it was shortlisted for a Mind Media Award and Michelle has shown it in a range of settings including at a Royal College of Psychiatrists conference. Michelle hopes that the film will be a springboard for her ambition to make a longer film about a young woman developing a psychosis: something which happened to her.

Michelle in her own words

As Gordon McManus said in my film *Recovery*, once you have the awareness that you are mentally ill and confront it, you can begin your journey of recovery. I think everyone's journey is unique. You have to work at it. It's not easy when you are experiencing symptoms and the effects of medication. You can feel isolated and prefer to have a routine rather than try new things. Cognitive behavioural therapy (CBT) really helped me confront these fears and grow as a person as a result.

Making the *Recovery* film has made a huge impact on my life. I thought at points that I did not have it in me to produce a piece of work that would make a difference to people's lives. Some of the film mirrored my own experiences; people were sectioned and hospitalised and that sort of thing and I know what it's like to be in hospital, I know what it's like to be very unwell.

My objective was to produce a piece of work that everyone could watch and learn something about mental illness. Although there are no mental healthcare professionals in the film itself, I was supported by my psychologist while I was making the film, and now it is being used as a teaching tool to promote 'recovery' throughout the South London and Maudsley NHS Foundation Trust.

Both Jerome Carson and I have talked about sending copies of the film to recovery centres in other parts of the world, particularly the USA, Australia and New Zealand. However, we have no budget at the moment. My hope is that the trust will help to make this happen.

The four participants in the *Recovery* film certainly seemed pleased about the way they were portrayed. Gordon said I was '*a pioneer*' and Dolly said I '*showed beautiful humanity in all of them*'. It was my intention all along to try and portray an honest account of their experiences of mental illness, to promote '*hope*' and '*belief that we can all lead a meaningful life*' as Gordon says.

One of the things that affected me a lot up until recently was the fact that I have lost so much time to mental illness that I am desperate to live and not miss out on any more opportunities that come my way. This has caused me to spread myself too thinly. I was aware that was happening and I talked to my family about this and they have offered me more support.

Apart from therapies and support from my family and friends, I work very hard at my own recovery. I have learned so much by listening about the experiences of other people. My work as a film-maker is also very important as it has offered me an outlet for my emotions. The *Recovery* film helped to unearth 'my demons' and still has an impact in how I approach my life. I used to hide my feelings to everyone before I became mentally ill. Now I talk about things that bother me. However, I do try and work through them myself. I now have a solid and loving relationship with my family and friends, which I did not have before I became mentally ill.

My next project is about a young girl who has a psychotic episode. This is a one-hour drama based on my own experiences. My hope is that it will help me find an 'agent' and gain me more exposure as a film-maker.

Michelle interviewed by Sarah

Michelle McNary is a woman who is recovering from schizophrenia and is a professional film-maker, who has just made a film about the recovery process. The film was a project funded by the Charitable Trustees of the South London and Maudsley NHS Foundation Trust, and proved so good that it was nominated for a Mind Media Award competing alongside the BBC and Channel 4.

This film is unique in involving service users on both sides of the camera. This shared experience of mental illness, Michelle feels, put her in a 'privileged position' and helped her to understand what the interviewees were going through. She says, '*Some of it mirrored my own experience. People were sectioned and hospitalised and that sort of thing and I know what it's like to be in hospital, I know what it's like to be very unwell.*'

So she had an empathy with her participants, which might explain why the four people featured in the film were portrayed so positively. However, it wasn't just the film that gained from the people involved, Michelle benefited from it as well. She personally found their stories inspiring and she explains, '*They helped me analyse what recovery was and realise my own life and how I could make my own recovery better.*'

You would think with a nomination from Mind, alongside stalwarts such as the BBC and Channel 4, Michelle is a past master at documentary making, but amazingly this is her first attempt, although she did watch '*quite a few*' films before embarking on the project.

The film focuses on four individuals' views on recovery and for Michelle the theme of hope that is presented is '*fundamental, absolutely fundamental*' to the recovery process. She adds that belief is also important. She says, '*I think they're the same thing in a sense. Because if you don't think things are going to get any better, then why would you bother to do what you're doing? .... You wouldn't feel inspired to, would you?*'

She was committed to presenting a positive piece of work. She admits the thing she maybe didn't focus on was '*how hard it is for the day-to-day living sometimes, but I didn't want to focus on the negative. I was focusing on the positive. Look forward, don't look back.*' She thinks that living a meaningful life is important, as Gordon McManus says himself in the film.

The content of the film is heart wrenching at points and I ask Michelle if there were any emotional points for her? She volunteers that, '*A couple of things James said about how he'd like to be an established author, but it's probably a pipe dream.... That made me sad,*' but she continues, '*essentially the film is really uplifting and positive and there aren't really any sad moments.*'

Of course she was 'very happy' to be short-listed for the Mind awards, '*against Beebs, Channel 4 and all that. I was really pleased. I got a bit of recognition at last, you know.*' She admits that she was disappointed that she didn't win anything but she adds modestly, '*I think I did quite well really.*' For a first documentary – just a bit.

After such a large project, she wants to embark on some shorter ones, but she intends to work on another big one focusing on the experience of psychosis. She says, '*It's really basically my life. This film is basically me, but with a younger person.*' She wants to open up the world of mental illness for more people to understand, but she stresses, '*Not all my films are going to be about mental illness*'.

She feels that film can help our understanding about recovery by showing '*people talking about their life*'. She feels, '*How they approach their own recovery is going to definitely help other people.*' She believes it gives people a guide. She enthuses, '*I mean they can be inspired by people like Dolly, James, Gordon and Ben and* [Ben Haydon is one of the four who featured in Michelle's *Recovery* film] *see what they've done in their lives that has helped them.*'

The participants certainly seemed pleased about the way they were portrayed. Michelle confides: '*Well, this might sound a bit egotistical actually, but Gordon turned round and said I was a pioneer* [she laughs] *apparently. Dolly said I showed beautiful humanity in all of them.*' No award perhaps, but plenty of praise. This is crucial for Michelle, she says: '*I thought well if they liked it, well I've done my job.*'

It's receiving attention from the world of psychiatry as well, as Michelle gave two presentations at the annual meeting of the Social and Rehabilitation Section of the Royal College of Psychiatrist's conference in Bristol. If you needed any more evidence of the energy Michelle has invested in this project, this talk was in fact two talks about recovery back to back. Michelle says, '*Their reaction was really, really positive. A lot of them said that they would contact Dan Charlton about getting copies, and we're trying to get it out to all the trusts, not just London.*' Not content with the whole of London, she says, '*It's also going to be at festivals.*' The South London and Maudsley Trust are going to help in this area as well.

After standing alongside the work of major TV channels, she is now hoping to get the film on the BBC and Channel 4. The idea is to '*use it as a bench mark for my own future directing work*'. There's no stopping this woman, she's after an agent so she can '*see what happens there*'.

Yet she's far from exhausted. She even hopes to start a *Recovery* film club. When she was actually making the film she describes how she'd get up and do her editing in the morning till nine. And here she reveals what kept her going: '*I got up every morning absolutely looking forward to the day. I absolutely did. I loved every minute of it. It was hard at points. Technically it was challenging and creatively it was challenging, but I have to say I woke up every morning in a great mood thinking what am I going to do today?*'

She is aware that, '*It did take over most of my life, but then most people's work does.*' As much as she enjoyed it, now that it's done she finds it '*a bit of a relief. I mean it is tiring and demanding doing editing. I don't think I could have carried on like that forever or anything like that. But it was fun while it lasted. I really enjoyed it a lot.*'

This is the start rather than the end for Michelle. She wants to move onto still larger projects '*and just keep making films*'. And crucially for her, '*It helps me recover doing my work like the people in my film talk about how important they're creativity is to their recovery and I feel exactly the same way*'.

For Michelle, a recovery hero is anyone who achieves anything while on medication, and dealing with all the side effects of medication and symptoms. However, though she says of others, '*they should be the heroes, they're the people who are getting through the day*', but when it comes to whether she considers herself a hero, she simply says: '*I'd like to think so*', but she doesn't think about it that way.

She laughs at the suggestion that she has become a bit of a campaigner saying, '*Well maybe. I'm not a dogmatic type of person.... But if people were inspired by my work and it helps them in some way that's marvellous.*'

An appraisal of Michelle by Jerome

The *Recovery* film was one of the most important projects I have ever been involved in within my entire professional career. My role within this process is best described in Carson (2011) and the full background to the film and its participants and origins can be seen in Carson *et al* (2008). Without Michelle, there would have been no *Recovery* film. To see the film go to: www.slam.nhs.uk/patients/recovery.aspx (accessed July 2011).

Russell Guthrie from the trust communications department and myself accompanied Michelle and her family to the Mind Media Awards in November 2010, for which Michelle had been nominated. The event was hosted by Lord Melvin Bragg and John Sergeant, the former BBC political correspondent. Sitting in this very 'plush' cinema in the South Bank, London, as we went through the various award categories, I felt incredibly privileged just to be there. In Michelle's category, 'New Media', Michelle was up against the BBC and Channel Four, a real David versus Goliath battle. Not surprisingly, she did not win on this occasion, but sitting there it struck me as ironic that Michelle's film was probably the only film that was made by someone with a major mental disorder. You might think that a charity such as Mind, the voice of the mental health sufferer, might have recognised this by giving her a special award.

Michelle's *Recovery* film is significant for a number of reasons. First, she presents the four people featured as '*philosophers of recovery*'. Second, it is a film rather than just four people talking in front of the camera, which is the case with many so-called recovery films on YouTube. Third, making it has helped Michelle learn a lot more about recovery. As her personal psychologist for a number of years, it was always my feeling that making the film would teach Michelle more about her own personal journey of recovery than I ever could. Lastly, the film is a wonderful recovery training resource, which I am sure will inspire countless people across the globe. Those of us who have tried to introduce recovery focused approaches into services will always be indebted to Michelle for her huge achievement in making such a memorable film.

Conclusion

In making a film about recovery, Michelle took the biggest step in her own recovery journey. She had to devise a budget for the film, select a producer, audition potential participants, direct and shoot the film, and then she spent 18 months editing the film herself. The end result, her *Recovery* film, has had much critical acclaim not least for the way she has presented the film's four central characters all of whom have been diagnosed with psychosis. Michelle now hopes she can make a film about a young woman with psychosis. Her own real life story.

References

Carson J, Holloway F, Wolfson P & McNary M (2008) (Eds) *Recovery Journeys: Stories of coping with mental health problems*. London: South London and Maudsley NHS Foundation Trust.

Carson J (2011) *Recovery: The long and winding road that leads to....* In: H Cordle, J Fradgley, J Carson, F Holloway & P Richards (2011) (Eds) *Psychosis Stories of Recovery and Hope*. London: Quay Books.

Chapter 11

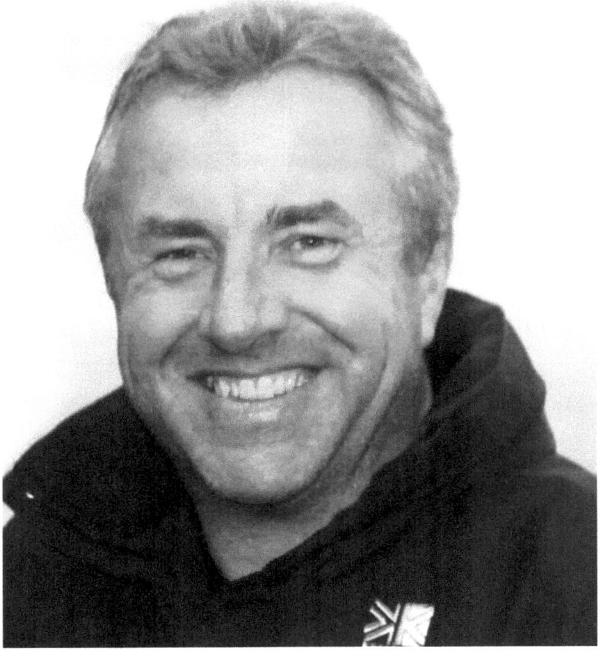

Stuart Baker-Brown

Summary

Stuart was diagnosed with schizophrenia and was told he was one of the worst cases the services had encountered. Being put on the wrong medication led to major weight gain. Encountering a befriender, which is a person who agrees to become a 'friend' to a person with a disability, and getting the right medication persuaded him to do something truly ambitious, which was to show that schizophrenia could be overcome. With the help of a Churchill Travelling Fellowship he climbed to Everest Base

Camp. He has given many presentations since, which have been illuminated by the amazing photographs he has taken on his travels. He has also been very prominent in campaigns to tackle stigma and discrimination against people with mental health problems.

Stuart in his own words

Schizophrenia took its strongest grip on me after I had visited the USSR in August 1991. During my visit I took part in marching on the streets of Moscow against communist hardliners, who attempted a coup against the then Russian leader Mikhail Gorbachev. When I returned to London I started to feel very anxious about the situation I had just returned from and became concerned about possible persecution from the KGB.

I fell into a world of anxiety and fear and believed the secret services were not only going to harm me physically but were trying to destroy me with the use of telekinetic/psychic powers. Little did I know the long destructive journey I was about to take. Nor did I understand the creation of the man who would unfold in the future.

Since my condition was triggered I have been on a 'quest' for greater understanding of all I have been through. My diagnosis is a correct diagnosis. I have experienced voices, psychosis, thought disorder, suicidal thoughts, depression, lack of motivation, the feeling of being controlled by outside forces and fear of persecution.

I am constantly in search for the possible truth behind my own symptoms, such as believing the KGB were harming me through psychic activity, the process of remote viewing. Or believing I could stumble across the random codes of the universe and was in contact with the Gods. I also had the ability to mentally time travel and experience contact with my past and future self. I shared my mind with other consciousnesses.

Although disabling, my condition has also been very intriguing and taught me much. I now believe we know very little of who and what we truly are, or the space we occupy, and the space we don't occupy. Schizophrenia has taught me that reality is an individual experience, an individual perception of the world which surrounds us and my reality is unique to me, as any individual's reality is unique to them. Although, in so many ways we are all the same, our experience and perception of life is separate and I believe this needs to be respected.

My path has been very long and destructive. Some years ago I cried at the thought of shaving. I had nothing to live for and any ambition was taken away from me, not only by my diagnosis but by those who surrounded me. My physical journey has also been devastating. In 1996 when I was first diagnosed, I weighed 94kg. Four years later I weighed 162kg. I have also been diagnosed with type 2 diabetes. Incorrect medication can be disastrous.

Death sometimes was the only way forward, an escape and an option that stayed with me for many years. My life was ruled by voices, the Scotsman, the penetrating eyes and scornful words of my mother. For many years I did not wear a watch, I did not feel part of time or part of the human race.

Schizophrenia takes away the ability to function in normal life. The condition has knocked my confidence and left me feeling worthless. The ability to work, have a mortgage, create a family and have the right to live a normal life has been taken from me not only by the condition but by others and the demoralising and degrading way they view my diagnosis.

Acceptance of my situation was key to my recovery. Over the years I became my own best doctor and began to learn about my own symptoms, the potential triggers and how to deal with these symptoms. Many years ago I fought to get these images and feelings out of my head, but the more I fought with symptoms the stronger they often became. Once I learnt to understand and accept my experiences, the weaker, for example, the voices became and the more control I gained.

In recent years I have changed my perception of my diagnosis and although my life has been a tumultuous journey full of devastation, it has also been a journey of self-discovery. Without my condition, I may have never climbed and trekked in the Himalayas. I for sure would have never achieved what I have achieved in the media and would have never been awarded a Winston Churchill Fellowship or other awards for my work fighting stigma and discrimination towards mental illness. Schizophrenia has given me a purpose.

Although I neither have the strength nor the will to experience my past again, my path has helped to open my mind and come to the understanding about the possibilities of the unseen and the unknown. Schizophrenia has broadened my outlook. Although I still face many difficulties, I am at a place I never thought I would reach. My type 2 diabetes has disappeared and I am currently a fit man weighing 98kg. The one thing which has always kept me going is a personal belief in me!

I am far from the man who was told by psychiatry he was one of the most severe undiagnosed cases of schizophrenia they had come across. A man who once accused his ex-wife of being a KGB spy placed to keep an eye on him.

Schizophrenia has made me who I am. I have come through not only personal pain but a life changing experience that has turned me into, I hope, a much more insightful and compassionate man.

Stuart interviewed by Sarah

Stuart Baker-Brown is a mental health activist diagnosed with schizophrenia. In the time since his diagnosis he has climbed Everest and has been the public face for the Time to Change campaign. However, things for him have not always seemed so positive.

Stuart says his schizophrenia was fully triggered in 1991 when he went to march in Moscow at the time that Communist hardliners were trying to overthrow Gorbachev. He has very vivid memories of the beginning of this process. He says, '*on the second day of marching I felt it was quite a tense situation and when I was in the hotel room asleep I got a call about 2.00am ... and there was just this bloke talking to me in Russian and I picked up only bits of his conversation. It was basically "What the hell are you doing?" and "Who the hell are you to get involved in our politics?" I put the phone down and straight away I felt very threatened, my heart started pounding and I became quite fearful.*'

This was the beginning of paranoia that would lead him to hearing command voices and experiencing hallucinations. He went to his GP in London after he experienced what he says was his worst psychotic experience.

But the paranoia that had caused him to seek help in the first place was also what drove him away from the psychiatric profession, believing they may be linked to the secret services. This time he uprooted himself and went to live in Exmoor.

Stuart says he thinks he saw a psychiatrist in Devon and a family GP. He tells me, '*Although schizophrenia was mentioned it wasn't diagnosed, but all they basically came up with was they wanted me to go into a psychiatric unit on a voluntary basis. The GP suggested that a few times and he also suggested electro convulsive therapy (ECT)*'. He had refused treatment because his best friend's father had a lot of mental health issues and Stuart had been brought up with how '*horrific*' ECT was and how '*awful*' the psychiatric units were. He says, '*they weren't exactly a place where you improved in life, in fact they made you worse. So I just didn't want to get involved with psychiatric units or ECT.*' Eventually he became house bound on the edge of Exmoor '*trying to deal with everything myself.*'

Of hearing voices, he says, '*I found that they became very strong in life the more stressed I was, I think what the voices were, and also all the symptoms that I've experienced of schizophrenia were issues from the past. All the stress within me was coming out as a sort of psychosis, because I was never one for really talking about my issues in the past. I don't get it anymore because I've learnt to really express myself. Stress has to come out in some way and some people turn to drink, some people turn to drugs, and for me psychosis was lifelong pressure suddenly releasing itself as stress.*'

The turn around he felt came when he started taking Seroquel. He says, '*within a few weeks of being on Seroquel I completely changed because it was controlling my symptoms. As it sedated me, I got a good night's sleep.*' He is very clear in his own mind that he doesn't think it took away the voices, but he says, '*that was me that dealt with that, but the medication did calm me down.*'

He experienced worse symptoms on previous medications, he says, '*I was having horrific nightmares, I was shaking, I had Parkinson-type symptoms. My ex-wife would tell you I couldn't hold a cup of coffee, I would just spill it, and on one occasion I held up a spoon to her and I just burst into tears because I didn't know it was a spoon and I was suffering memory loss as well, and I was told by the psychiatric team this is schizophrenia, but within three weeks of changing medication the nightmares began to stop.*'

For him the beginning of his recovery was dealing with the symptoms, he says, '*being able to sleep not having nightmares, feeling better within myself ... at first it was a mental thing, then once I began to feel better mentally, recovery went on to now I've got to recover my body and start losing weight.*'

Once his mental recovery had started, his campaigning began, motivated by what he described as his '*diabolical treatment*' on the NHS. He is quick to praise the NHS for the physical treatment he has received over the years, but he says, '*when you're dealing with mental health and psychiatry it's a completely different ball game*'. When he was recovering he was looking for stories of people who had recovered and gone on to do great things and there was nothing. He was dismayed, and said that *'everybody around me, the psychiatric team, everybody, was telling me that this was my life – you're not going to recover ... I just knew that I didn't want anyone to go through what I'd been through ... because of the negative impact it had on me. It wasn't right, it wasn't fair.'*

His journey of recovery began in 2001. *'I'd had three very lucky breaks around about 2001. The first was meeting the befriender who was very encouraging towards me, and the second was when I was put on Seroquel, which really worked for me ... so I was feeling very positive and the third was as I began to feel so positive I started to look into big things I could do to help other people who experienced psychosis or schizophrenia. I said I wanted to do something really big that was going to promote recovery and he* [the befriender] *suggested to me that he had a friend who had a Winston Churchill travel fellowship and he encouraged me to try for that.'* Stuart wanted to get to Everest Base Camp, do the trek, and use it as a symbol for overcoming schizophrenia. He says, *'I used to call it mount schizophrenia, Everest'*.

Stuart approached the fellowship drastically overweight with no real expectation of being accepted and as he recounts, he kept getting through to the next selection round until they said to him, *'We believe you can do it'* and that helped him really get away from psychiatry because as he explains, *'I thought hang on, there's these really influential, real powerful people you know in the country all telling me I could do this, they believed in me ... suddenly I had the Churchill Trustees saying, go for it and we'll support you and that was a huge confidence boost.'*

The trek was no picnic and he did it with a very high prescription of antipsychotics, which exacerbated altitude sickness. He admits, *'I was quite unwell and I did become sort of delusional at times,'* but he reached Everest Base Camp despite these obstacles.

He didn't end his campaigning there. He then went on to feature in an advert for the Time to Change campaign called *'Schizo'* shown in 2010 in nearly 2,000 cinemas across the UK. Time to Change hired an advertising team to do something about schizophrenia and Stuart was asked to do it, he says, *'I just sort of fitted the bill really.'*

He says, *'What I hoped to achieve was people would see someone with schizophrenia who looks normal, who is speaking normally and is doing something good like standing in front of a camera and giving a positive message.'*

When asked about what he considers to be his greatest achievement, Stuart responded, '*I don't think I've achieved it yet*'. He finds the hardest thing to deal with is not his illness but the attitude that the label evokes in people. He says, '*the reason I was ashamed of schizophrenia was not because I was ashamed, it was because other people made me feel ashamed about it.*' Now he says, '*I see it as a part of me, it's a side of me, it's everything that makes up Stuart Baker-Brown.*'

'*Do I see myself as a recovery hero? That's for other people to judge. I think a recovery hero is somebody who has got the guts to stand up and inspire other people, people who have risen above expectations forced upon them by others.*'

An appraisal of Stuart by Jerome

I have met Stuart on two separate occasions. The first was when he spoke at our psychosis conference. Linden Lynn, the co-editor of a book called *Beyond the Storms* (2008), wrote some of the following notes about his presentation:

'*Stuart ... was undiagnosed partly due to his inability to engage with services, because of his extreme sensitivity and withdrawal.... Stuart described himself as physically vortexed into my own dark mind.... He was shocked by the despondent attitudes he encountered (among staff).... He selected to climb to Mount Everest Base Camp as a symbolic and significant journey of recovery.*'

Stuart showed a number of the photographs that he took on his Everest expedition (see www.stuartbakerbrown.com) which made an incredibly engaging presentation.

The second time I met Stuart was at the Royal Society. He was there for the launch of Health Talk Online's new page on psychosis (see www.healthtalkonline.org under 'schizophrenia' and not 'psychosis'). After the formal presentations we discussed his Churchill Travelling Fellowship, which he was awarded in 2002 and he used this to travel to Everest Base Camp.

Stuart also featured in two Time to Change videos (2010). The one mentioned in his interview with Sarah was the '*Schizo*' cinema advert (this can be accessed via the Time to Change website, www.time-to-change.org.uk). This is a very striking film that has a scary beginning and just as a door opens you see Stuart standing making a cup of tea in a beautiful, bright and airy kitchen. He looks to the camera and says the following:

'Hi there! I'm sorry to disappoint you if you were expecting to see a lunatic with a knife on some sort of rampage. My name is Stuart and I was diagnosed with schizophrenia 12 years ago. People like me with a diagnosis of schizophrenia face stigma and discrimination every day. Luckily for me, I have the support of friends and family who help me lead a full life.'

A second film on the website is entitled, *Schizophrenic Man Terrifies Kids at a Party* and shows Stuart playing games with children very naturally at a party.

Stuart has also written a lot about his condition with a feature on the BBC News webpage entitled, *A Beautiful Mind* (2007). There is also an article on his travels in the Himalayas on the online journal *Irked Magazine* (2009).

One of the things that Stuart looked for in vain when he was first given the diagnosis of schizophrenia was '*stories of people who had recovered and have gone on to do great things.*' His own story is now adding to a series of service user accounts that can truly inspire and give hope to sufferers and their families and that may change the despondent attitudes of staff.

Conclusion

Like many people, Stuart's initial encounters with mental health services were not very positive. His recovery involved the right medication, having a befriender who encouraged him and having the ambition to travel to Nepal to climb to Everest Base Camp. The Churchill Trustees believed in his vision in a way that many mental health professionals might not have done, and awarded him a Travelling Fellowship. Since then, he has been involved in several public awareness campaigns to raise consciousness about mental health and to break down the barriers of stigma and discrimination.

References

BBC (2007) A Beautiful Mind [online]. Available at: http://news.bbc.co.uk/1/hi/magazine/7037314.stm (accessed July 2011).

Davidson L & Lynn L (2009) *Beyond the Storms: Reflections on personal recovery in Devon*. Exeter: Devon Partnership NHS Trust.

Health Talk Online (2011) [online]. Available at: www.healthtalkonline.org (accessed July 2011).

Irked Magazine (2009) [online]. Available at: www.irkedmagazine.com (accessed July 2011).

Stuart Baker-Brown [online]. Available at: www.stuartbakerbrown.com (accessed July 2011).

Time to Change campaign (2011) [online]. Available at: www.time-to-change.org.uk (accessed July 2011).

Chapter 12

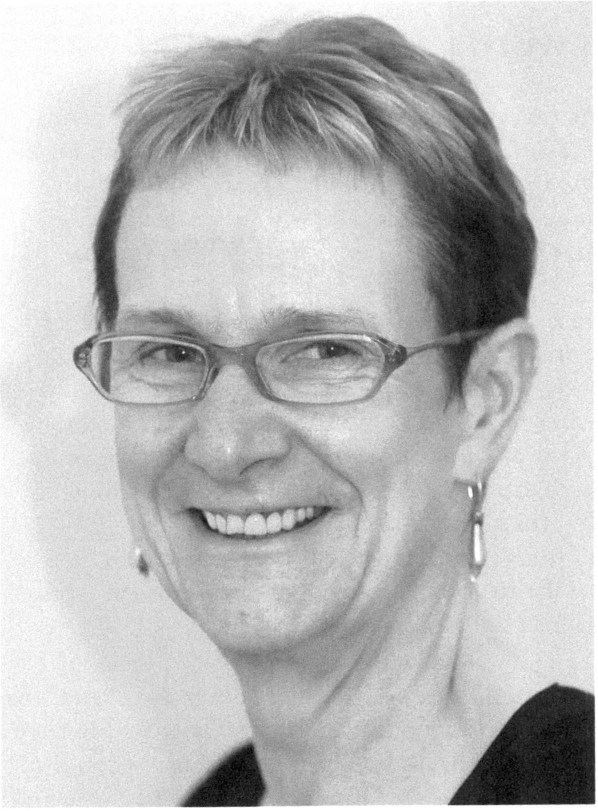

Rachel Perkins

Summary

Rachel Perkins is one of the most dynamic clinical psychologists in Britain. She was awarded an OBE for her services to mental health, especially in the employment field. In this chapter she talks about her three psychiatric careers and tells us that she has just started her fourth. As detailed in her chapter *My Three Psychiatric Careers* (1999) her careers have been as a clinical psychologist, a service user, a mental health activist, and now as the Chair of Equality 2025.

Rachel in her own words

Until 2010 I had three psychiatric careers: I had worked in mental health services for 30 years, written about them for 25 years and used them for 20 years. The first career was one that I applied for, the second I elected to do, the third was thrust upon me (see Perkins (1999) for a fuller description of Rachel's three psychiatric careers).

My first psychiatric career took me from being an Assistant Psychologist at Broadmoor Special Hospital via clinical training at the Institute of Psychiatry, and then I progressed through to Clinical Psychology to Clinical Director of Rehabilitation. I then went onto general adult mental health services and on to being Director of Quality Assurance and User Experience in South West London. Throughout, I was drawn to those people whom most services had written off – those 'chronic patients' who despite the ministrations of experts of all hues had failed to get better and who had historically been consigned to the back wards of remote asylums (in whose demise I played a role for the first part of my career).

I rapidly learned who the real experts were. To be sure, I saw the casualties of our system – people on whom services had given up and who had in turn given up on themselves and their possibilities. But among those whom I had the privilege to serve, I also found the most amazing wealth of courage, creativity and ingenuity in surviving, and thriving, in the face of what seemed to me like insurmountable odds. I soon realised the limitations of all the therapies I had been taught. I began to question the whole clinical paradigm 'treatment and cure', whether couched in organic, psychological or systemic terms. Most people I met wanted a life not a psychologist, and the extent to which the psychological therapy could assist in this ambition was limited. I am not saying that treatment has no place, but I became convinced that a focus on the reduction and elimination of deficits and dysfunctions was a woefully inadequate framework for understanding the challenges people face and assisting them in rebuilding their lives.

My concerns about the limitations of clinical paradigms became even more acute when I became a mental patient myself. I felt completely at sea without map or compass, amazed at how little my professional training helped me to navigate life with mental health problems. It was not until I spent some time in the USA in the early 1990s that I found a way of thinking about mental health conditions that made sense to me as both provider and recipient of mental health services. I met amazing people like Judi Chamberlin and Patricia Deegan and was introduced to ideas about recovery: an approach born not from learned professionals, but from the lived experience of people who had themselves faced the challenge of living with and growing beyond a diagnosis of mental health problems.

Recovery turns all of the traditional approaches on their head. Mental health services move from centre stage to the wings. In the foreground is our journey – where we have been, what has happened to us, where we are now, what we have got going for us and where we want to get to in life. Mental health professionals do not hold the key – the question is whether we can be of any assistance at all in people's journey. Treatment is not centre stage – it is in the margins. Getting rid of problems (by whatever means) is neither necessary nor sufficient for getting back a life. Instead the essence of the journey that is recovery revolves around making sense of what has happened, recognising your own resources and resourcefulness, and having fertile ground in which you can grow within and beyond what has happened to you. Hope is critical, as are taking back control and having the opportunity to do the things you value and participate as an equal citizen. As Mary O'Hagan has said – mental health professionals are *'carriers of technologies that we may want to use at times, just like architects, plumbers and hairdressers,'* (O'Hagan, 2007).

I became less and less satisfied with my role as clinical psychologist, and if I wanted to change the experience and opportunities of those whom I served, I had to change whole service systems. So I went feral: I became a director – I started setting up new initiatives like employing people with lived experience of mental health problems in mental health services and trying to make the service where I worked more recovery focused. An important lesson I had learned was that people who have walked a similar path are often our most important travelling companions and can offer the gift of hope and images of possibility, inspire in us the courage to face the challenges that lie along the way.

But I learned one more thing back in the USA. I learned that we are part of a larger movement – the movement of disabled people. I saw how a social model of disability made sense in understanding the challenges that we all face: we are not disabled by our impairments (mobility, sensory, cognitive or emotional). We are disabled by the way in which society fails to accommodate us but instead devalues us, marginalises and excludes us. I learned how a language of rights offers a more empowering and liberating framework than that of individual deficits, dysfunctions and needs.

It was in the civil rights movement that ideas about recovery were born. It is by replacing ideas about 'needs' with ideas about rights that we can move, in the words of my partner Liz Sayce, from psychiatric patient to citizen. Not just rights to treatment and support, but those positive rights: to live independently, participate on equal terms in all facets of life and have control over our destiny and the support/treatment we receive. It is alongside our peers with physical impairments, learning disabilities and long-term health conditions that we can best achieve those rights. There have been gains made: legislation outlawing discrimination on the grounds of disability and affording us the rights to those adjustments and supports we require to live as equal citizens. But while there may be 10 miles behind us, there are 10 thousand more to go in making equal citizenship a reality.

So in 2010, I retired from my first psychiatric career (not the second or third) and embarked on a fourth. At the time of writing I have been appointed Chair of Equality 2025, which is the cross-government strategic advisory group on issues relating to disabled people, and I am involved in work on disability hate crimes, right to control, the work capability assessment, disability employment programmes ... and much more. I have not completely abandoned the ambition to change mental health services – I am still working on the project team for the Implementing Recovery – Organisational Change programme – but my aim is to pursue the rights and opportunities of those of us with mental health conditions as part of a broader disability rights agenda. So watch this space.

Rachel interviewed by Sarah

Rachel Perkins is one of those rare psychologists that have been on both sides of the mental health fence. She refers to it as her three psychiatric careers, as a clinical psychologist, as a patient and as a mental health activist.

She is reticent in saying that she has learnt more from any of these '*careers*', instead she says, '*I suppose it's difficult to ascribe learning to any one of them. I mean I'd have to say all of them, because working in mental health services allows you to meet hundreds of people who live the most amazing lives and whose reality is often very different from that which other people share. So I guess I learned huge amounts from the clients, who I've had the privilege to serve in the mental health services over the years, but obviously I've also learned a great deal from my own lived experience.*'

She is very clear that each person has their unique own journey. She says, '*In a sense I suppose, what I found most shocking about it* [her own mental health difficulties] *was it really did seal for me just how little professionals know about living a life with a mental health condition, that it was amazing how little being a clinical psychologist helped me to navigate life with a mental health condition.*'

With regards to the psychologist career she has retired from, she says she has become, '*increasingly dissatisfied with a kind of clinical gaze for looking at mental health issues*'. She says, '*Over the last 10 or 15 years I've been doing a lot of work in the broader disability rights arena … I'd like to see mental health services really on a sort of periphery somewhere.*'

She was attracted to the American Civil Rights inspired, '*rights rather than needs paradigm*' as she finds it a much more '*empowering and liberating way of thinking about what people need in order to live as equal citizens*'. So this is what she says she has decided to spend the last bit of her career doing.

For her this seems to have been a natural progression, she thought she would have regrets after working in the same place for 23 years, but she says, '*I haven't missed it for a day*'. And she is still involved in mental health services on the Implementing Recovery, Department of Health funded programme and as chair of Equality 2025, the cross-government advisory group on issues affecting disabled people.

She is happy to use the term 'disabled' because like the broader disability movement she adopts a social model of disability: problems do not lie in the individual but in the form of barriers in society, by the way in which a society '*fails to accommodate us but instead excludes us, denies us rights, so what is disabling is the world in which we live*'. She is very emphatic on this point.

Rachel refuses to get bogged down in debates about terminology. She asserts that, '*any language creates traps. There's been just as many criticisms of the term recovery.*'

One of her few pauses for thoughts comes from the enquiry about when she was first ill, after which she says, '*I was first properly diagnosed about 21 years ago, but while I'd been at university, I'd sort of had various prescriptions for antidepressants, my GP had told me to take long walks and all this idiot sort of things, so I suppose there was a period when...*' she pauses again, '*...you know, life was fairly stormy, but I didn't have a formal diagnosis. I wasn't given a formal diagnosis or admitted to hospital until 21 years ago*'. She attributes all the things that she can do and says, '*to me that includes manic depression as much as I attribute the bad bits of my life*'.

Although in the case of her diagnosis she does feel that it shifted something. She says, '*I suppose becoming one of "them" not "one of us" and living for the next forever on the sort of no man's land between them and us is, I think, it's quite an exciting place to live actually. I feel sorry for people who don't experience the extremes of life.*' And she feels it has made her better at what she does. She qualifies, '*I mean I'm not doing some sort of cutesy "everything's lovely" kind of thing, because I hate being depressed, it's awful. But I don't think that all of the experiences that shape us and have value have to be pleasurable.*'

In terms of seeing her experiences as giving her a unique perspective, she is also quite wary as she says everyone's perspective is unique and so she doesn't consider herself special. '*I suppose there are ways in which I've been incredibly privileged in my life. I have faced the challenges that life's thrown at me, but I've had a hell of a foundation to face them on. I've had loads of opportunities to see and do loads of things, but I've also taken those opportunities.*'

She says, '*I think diagnosis means different things to different people. Some people find a diagnosis helpful, others hate it. You could say that manic depression is a genius disease and it's quite a good diagnosis to have and you know with its associations with creativity and the like. I think each person has to find a way of understanding the world that makes sense to them and allows them a way forward.*'

A friend of hers said that Rachel's recovery started when she realised that professionals didn't have the answers. She refused to romanticise her role: she hadn't dreamt of becoming a psychologist, but more happened to stumble upon it, because everyone had told her she wouldn't be able to cope with it. As for her own treatment approach, she says, *'I suppose I gave up treating people a long, long, time ago. Most people don't need therapy they need a life.'*

She is just as adamant about the importance of work in staying well. She says, *'In our society being paid for your contribution is the way in which we value that contribution – that means that there's a huge dignity in labour. One of the awful things that happens when you're marginalised as a "mental patient" is that, all of a sudden you end up on the receiving end of everybody else's good works, and there is no more horrible place to be'.*

To elaborate on this point she says, *'Somewhere to live, something to do and someone to love is actually a pretty good formula for what most of us need. So yes I think work is the thing that we're systematically excluded from'.*

It is hard to believe that she has any doubts, but she does say, *'I regularly doubt my ability to achieve anything ... Whether what I'm doing will achieve a fairer more inclusive world. I have absolutely no doubt that every human being is valuable and that every human being can contribute to the community in which they live ... But doubt how you get there, oh yeah, change my mind all the time. Develop and grow.'*

Tellingly she believes her greatest achievements were helping shut one of the old asylums, and all the work she has done in helping people to get and keep employment of their choice. She says, *'I am aware that some people don't like what I've done on employment, but I've seen more tears cried over getting the first pay cheque, than anything else'.*

Characteristically, she is hard to pin down on the definition of a recovery hero. *'I suppose my greatest difficulty with being interviewed is I don't know what a hero is. Maybe a hero is just someone who was in a place and a time and had a chance to make a difference.'*

She does say, *'I hope that throughout my career, what I've tried to do, is not get caught up in the doom and gloom ... You have to believe that there's a decent life possible.'*

But when asked directly if she considers herself as a hero, she says, *'No, I don't think anyone considers themselves a hero. Absolutely not.'*

An appraisal of Rachel by Jerome

I first met Rachel at a rehabilitation psychologists' training evening in the old District Services Centre at the Maudsley Hospital. As the assembled psychologists were waiting expectantly to hear the first speaker, a patient came into the room and lay on the floor near to the front of the room. One hundred of Britain's best rehabilitation psychologists sat glued to their seats! No one knew what to do. No one stirred. We all pretended the patient wasn't there! Rachel walked up to the patient and knelt down beside him. She whispered something to him, whereupon miraculously he got up and walked out of the room with her, and the conference was able to start. I was in awe of her after that episode! When I mentioned this to Rachel over 20 years later, with characteristic modesty she said that she had suggested the patient come with her and have a cup of tea, as he would only be bored listening to a group of psychologists. My next encounter was when I asked her to contribute a paper for a Special Issue of Clinical Psychology Forum, which I co-edited with Craig Newnes (Carson & Newnes, 1995). I was puzzled by the fact that at one stage I heard nothing from Rachel for over three months. I now realise she was probably unwell at this time. Some years later, I learned about her own struggles with mental illness, from the foreword to one of her books (Perkins & Repper, 1999). Indeed, for some years she wrote the service user column for the journal *Openmind*.

Rachel's views do not make either comfortable reading or listening for psychologists who believe in the importance of therapy. We invited her to speak to our Lambeth Recovery Group in February 2011, where in her presentation she talked about her non-belief in therapy. I did a quick head count of the audience and there were 29 people present, of whom 16 had received some therapy from me. Had we all been wasting our time? Rather than therapy, what people need she believes is '*somewhere to live, something to do and someone to love.*' Creating employment opportunities for people with mental health problems has been one of the major foci of her work. Interestingly this goes way back to work she published with Len Rowland in the late 1980s (Rowland & Perkins, 1988). In this regard, one of her greatest achievements was persuading the South West London and St George's NHS Foundation Trust to employ staff with lived experience of mental health problems. Without Rachel's vision, hundreds of people would not now be working in the NHS.

Rachel retired from the NHS in 2010, but as she points out, she is now involved with the wider movement on disability rights. I doubt she will go quietly in her retirement years.

Conclusion

Rachel is unique in having had three psychiatric careers. Having lived experience herself of severe mental health problems, she has tempered her views of what most helps sufferers. Her recipe for successful recovery is having somewhere to live, having something meaningful to do and having someone to love. It is humbling how many of the people who use our services do not possess these three key elements.

References

Carson J & Newnes C (Eds) (1995) Contemporary Perspectives in Psychiatric Rehabilitation. Special Issue of Clinical Psychology Forum; number 82.

O'Hagan M (2007) Parting thoughts from Mary O'Hagan. *Mental Notes September* **18** 4–5. New Zealand Mental Health Commission.

Perkins R (1999) *My Three Psychiatric Careers*. In: P Barker, P Campbell & B Davidson (Eds) *From the Ashes of Experience: Reflections on madness, survival and growth*. London: Whurr.

Perkins R & Repper J (1999) *Working Alongside People with Long Term Mental Health Problems*. London: Stanley Thornes.

Rowland L & Perkins R (1988) You can't eat, drink or make love eight hours a day: the value of work in psychiatry. *Health Trends* **20** 75–79.

Chapter 13

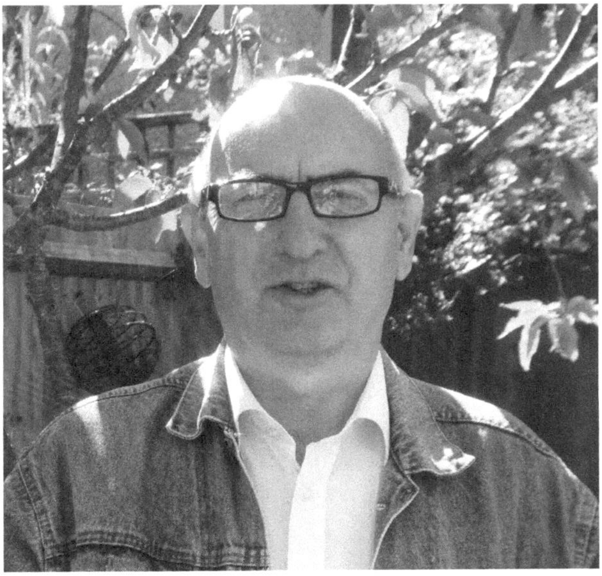

Andrew Voyce

Summary

Andrew describes his nomadic journey after failing to get a degree at university to years of revolving door admissions to mental hospital. He is grateful to Mrs Thatcher for closing down the old asylums and for developing the community care system, which has helped transform his life.

Andrew in his own words

Recovery is not like winning the lottery. It's not going to make everything OK. Look, I failed my final exams for my first university in 1974 but I got a

BA pass with the Open University (OU) in 1986. Where did that get me? It was the precursor to five years living on trains and in bus shelters, because the dear old health service had me still on an aversion therapy of mind bending and humiliating injections. As multiple times previously, I dropped them off and entered a world of signalling, mesmeric isolation, a certainty that the Soviets were coming, that the IRA were lurking on caravan sites and Kentish lanes, a whole load of unhelpful things. It's hard, but you can be detained and medicated for your own good and for the good of your objects of mainly victimless crime, so named. You can come out the other end. I emerged and was not on injections. I was together enough to be able to use those windows of awareness, which at first occurred only for a short time each day to obtain an BA Honours from the OU and then a Master of Arts in Social and Public Policy from Brighton University. I emerged from residential home to group home and eventually to an individual flat. I was Andrew Voyce MA. But why bother? Sure if you have my predispositions to be able to work hard and purposefully at academia, you can get at the age of almost 50 what should have been arranged by the caring services at 30. It could have been a life changing attribute at 30, but at age 50 it just showed what a waste of time asylum life was, now thankfully no more, due to Mrs Thatcher's well considered decimation of those pernicious institutions. Was it worth the trouble?

It's not exactly the make up of a recovery hero. No sir. I hear that six months into employment, the average MA holder is earning £29k per annum. Hold on there, 12 years after the award ceremony, I'm just creeping onto permitted earnings and am 99% supported by the state.

So the academic issues are there, if they are of value to the average member of the public. I laboured for years under the allusion of Keynesian economics, which provided me with a non-devalued A-level at grade B in 1969, and first year university pass in 1970. This allusion was that it was in the gift of government to cure unemployment. I hung onto this belief, as doubtless did many others, and indeed as a worker in the City of London during the 1983 election, I wore a red tie to work! My MA studies taught me that in fact inflation can be controlled by interest rates, so goodbye Keynesian misconceptions! Hello Chancellor Gordon Brown and the independent Bank of England, the Monetary Policy Committee and 10 years of low inflation – a blessing to those on low incomes, myself included.

I could not have understood that without my MA. But do I now need to study why it is that inflation is roaring away again yet interest rates are at record lows? Is there some new paradigm? Should I have bothered at all? It all gives you a sense of perspective.

I firmly believe that mental health service user views of all sorts should be accepted as part of everyone's life. We need to have a culture that includes service user narrative; a culture that embraces the disparate ways that reality can be perceived.

Finally, can you believe that all this has happened to me, that I've had to deal with challenges to the wisdom taught to me at the highest levels? And it is in my hard wired consciousness alongside the conviction that after the time of the Helsinki Agreements that the Soviets were on their way here? And other unhelpful thoughts?

Andrew interviewed by Sarah

Andrew Voyce spent many years as a vagrant experiencing psychotic symptoms, but is now heavily involved in his community as a social entrepreneur after having completed an MA in social policy.

Despite his achievements Andrew has a lot of regrets about what he regards as 'unwise decisions' in his 20s, mainly involving drug taking and making bad financial choices.

'I got the compensation money from a bad road accident which I'd had at the age of 17. And it was enough to buy maybe one or two terraced houses in Reading at the time, and that's the sort of thing that working people spend all their lives paying off. I could have bought a house in Reading at the time and unfortunately I fell in with the wrong crowd and spent a lot of money on drugs.' He said at the time that he thought that *'the large sum of money that I got for compensation, it didn't really matter really what I did'*.

Later he was to lose a house when he was made redundant from a job in the city, through another, as he describes it, '*unwise decision*' of not paying his mortgage over this period of time. He says, *'I think that sort of unwise notion that I didn't have to pay the mortgage for two years, paralleled my actions when I got the compensation money when I was at Reading.'*

He says, *'I think my first episode followed a pattern of a predisposition towards being psychotic and I have severe bad life events: my road accident when I was 17, I lost a leg and that was quite a traumatic experience. When I was at Reading I took my final examinations, I sat my nine three-hour papers and I got the result of "fail" and that was quite a traumatic experience. And my parents got divorced, which was quite a traumatic experience. And also I spent a lot of my compensation money on smoking a lot of cannabis and taking LSD and things and I think that's proven nowadays to be a bad indicator for the onset of schizophrenia and psychosis, so in a way I think I followed a typical pattern.'*

Since being at his worst he has written a book called *The Durham Light* (Voyce, 2009) chronicling his experience. *'The period that I cover in that book 'The Durham Light' was from about 1986 to about 1991. A period of about five years and during that period I mainly was homeless and I slept in bus shelters and that, and I spent about two or three winters out in the wind and the snow in bus shelters and I was quite ill then, and that sort of epitomised the neglect which I experienced.'*

He had an extremely bad experience of the old asylums, but he managed to turn this around. He says, *'I was in hospital in 1991, I negotiated with the doctors and they didn't give me medication by injection, they gave me medication by tablet. I don't think I have missed a tablet hardly in the last 20 years since 1991, when I was last discharged, and I've lived in the community. I haven't been an inpatient, I haven't re-offended, I haven't lived as a vagrant. I've managed to pull my life around to many extents and I have more self-respect now. It's a pity that couldn't have been the case in 1974 when I was first admitted.'*

Today Andrew produces cartoons, poems and songs about his experiences and uses them as a positive and cathartic process. He doesn't consider himself angry, he says, *'I suppose I should be really, but I'm kind of sort of more philosophical, I'm very glad that the asylums have been closed down and it's strange to think that we've got Mrs Thatcher of all people to thank for closing those places down.'*

'I think getting better and hope and recovery are relative terms. They come along all of a sudden and you don't wake up one morning and think crikey, I'm better or crikey, recovery has arrived, you know I've got hope at last. You don't wake up one morning and these things happen, they sort of occur over a period of time ... hope I think is a state of mind and I don't have really any bad down sides to my life and I live in a nice flat in a housing association

property. It's got no rising damp, no window panes falling out, the boiler doesn't break down every winter. It's quite a nice place to live. I've got a lot of things going on in my life. I have activities in the mental health world … I'm a great believer in the power of narrative. It's therapeutic to create a narrative of your life in whatever shape or form, in written work either prose or poems. It helps to draw pictures and write songs around difficult times. That activity in itself can be very therapeutic.' He feels this creativity has helped to give him 'closure'.

Andrew has a very distinct idea of recovery, *'I would consider myself to be fully recovered if I could cobble together an independent lifestyle, where I wasn't dependent on benefits and support from the mental health world so much.'*

He feels his greatest achievement is his MA in social policy. He says, *'I've always had the potential to do that. It's a pity that I just had to endure 20 years as a revolving door patient rather than being got right and getting an MA in my 20s or 30s when it could have been a life changing event. I got it when I was almost 50, so it didn't turn out to be a life changing event.'*

He was encouraged to do the MA when he was discharged from hospital and he was awarded the MA from Brighton in 1998.

His hardest moment was being homeless and being in and out of the asylums, even at one point attempting suicide by overdosing on medication, which only gave him horrendous shakes. *'They were pretty grim times'*, he says.

Andrew says he has a sense of humour, but it's a black one, *'like saying I wonder if the nurses took bets on how long it would be before I was readmitted to the asylum when I was discharged. What do you say to a 20 year old experiencing their first episode of psychosis? – Don't worry you'll be all right when you're my age, 60.'* He laughs.

'I'd really very much like to lead the way, so to speak, amongst the people I know down here. This is a very backward part of the world, East Sussex. It's not like London at all, even though we're only 60 miles away. But I'm quite open to having a life after retirement age and it would be great if our social enterprise took off, if it became a means of earning a living, I would be quite open to that.'

There have certainly been successes in his projects as his personally made slide shows on life in the old asylums has gathered 6,500 hits on the internet.

His expectations for what a recovery hero is must be high, as he says, '*Well I think to be a proper recovery hero, I need to be moved on a stage further and whether I can do it at my present age with the resources that might come my way I wouldn't know.*'

As for thinking he is a recovery hero, he says, '*No I don't, as I say if I was going to be a role model I would have had to have done something to sort of be worthy of some of the things or some of the potential. I would have to be independent.*'

He says, '*I've maybe got tales of caution in a way. But I wouldn't have done the things I'm involved with today if I'd stayed in London for example*'. He finishes by saying, '*We live in a messed up society and it will mess up its people,*' but he doesn't see that as a reason to side step mental illness as an issue.

An appraisal of Andrew by Jerome

Andrew Voyce and I both attended Reading University. He failed his undergraduate degree and developed a major mental disorder. The fact that later on in life he went on to get both an undergraduate degree and a masters degree in social policy shows resilience of the highest order.

I first read about Andrew's story in an issue of *Mental Health Today*. I suggested to Hannah Cordle that we consider interviewing him for our new book on psychosis (Cordle *et al*, 2011). Andrew was one of the first people Hannah interviewed and I was very moved by this longer and more complete version of his story. He was the first of the contributors to this book to return his biography, though paradoxically one of the last to be interviewed.

In November 2010, I invited Andrew to speak at our local recovery group in South London. He did in fact give three separate presentations that afternoon. The first was the telling and sharing of his own personal story. The second was when he showed us a cartoon slide show of his life in the old asylum system (see www.slideshare.net/AndrewsAsylumLife). The third was when he talked us through a glossary of mental health terminology, covering issues such as advocacy and user involvement. He explained what each of these terms meant and his experience of them. Subsequently, I read his book, *The Durham Light*, which provides a captivating account of his 'years of madness'. Looking at him today dressed in a smart suit, it is hard to reconcile his current image with that of someone who lived such a disturbed nomadic life. His subsequent recovery is all the more remarkable. I think he now needs to write a book about his recovery and the steps he took to turn his life around so dramatically.

Conclusion

Andrew Voyce spent many years as a vagrant in the south of England after developing a major mental disorder. This period was punctuated with several admissions to the old asylums. The development of community care meant that Andrew's prospects were much improved and he went on to complete an undergraduate and masters degree. He has developed slideshows highlighting the inadequacies of the asylum model of care. His journey from '*revolving door schizophrenic*' to skilled presenter on mental health care is of heroic proportions.

References

Cordle H, Fradgley J, Carson J, Holloway F & Richards P (Eds) (2011) *Psychosis: Stories of recovery and hope*. London: Quay Books.

Voyce A (2009) *The Durham Light and Other Stories: A personal history of homelessness and schizophrenia*. London: Chipmunka.

Chapter 14

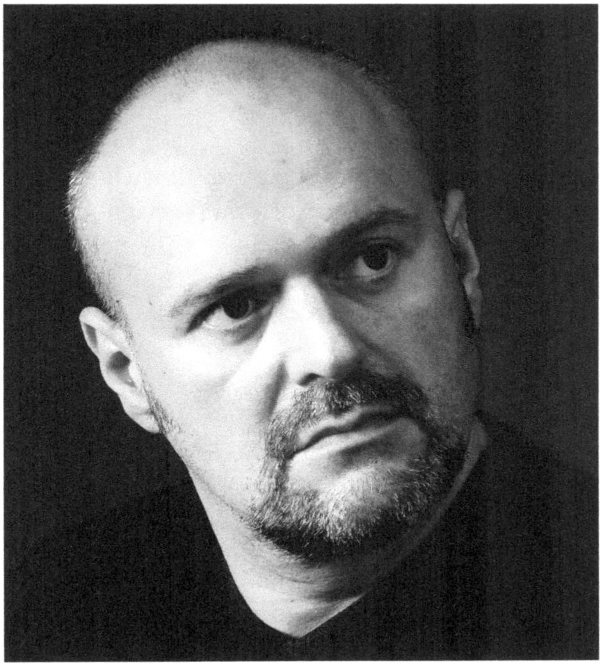

Matthew Ward

Summary

Matthew Ward was not diagnosed with bipolar disorder until he was 43. The diagnosis turned out to be life saving. He had suffered throughout his life with extreme mood swings and had made several attempts to take his life. His career as an actor helped protect him from some of the self-stigmatising effects of mental illness. He has been able to use his acting skills to help educate other service users, professionals, carers and the public about recovery.

Matthew in his own words

First of all, I want to state that I am not a recovery hero. It sounds like a nice title to have and the other individuals in this series are all worthy of that title, but I am not. I am a recovery survivor. My story is well documented in that I was not diagnosed with bipolar until I was 43, which is partly the stupidity of professionals, but also testament to my ability as an actor. I know that had I not been diagnosed and prescribed lithium, I would now be dead.

When I came to the Streatham team base, having disappeared with a plan to kill myself, I knew I had reached a moment where I would actually be successful in taking my own life or I would receive help. Over the years there had been many suicide attempts and disappearances, yet still I had not been diagnosed. This time I knew I just could not go on, it had to be sorted out one way or the other.

When I spoke to Davina Blunt, an occupational therapist at the team base, we both knew it was not just depression, and she recommended I see psychiatrist Dr McGowan who made a diagnosis of bipolar. It all seemed to make sense.

I have been one of the lucky ones. Lithium has taken the edge off my highs and lows. They are still there, but I am not as likely to give all my money away, sleep with complete strangers (female I hasten to add) or risk life and limb at the drop of a hat. I am more in control, although not totally in control (that would be boring), but more in control.

Through medication and the help I have received, I have my career back. I have put on a one-man play for Guy's and St Thomas's Charity Trust and I have given speeches on '*My recovery: A work in progress*' at conferences to service users and mental health care professionals alike. Using my acting ability and affinity with Shakespeare, hopefully I've given an insight into suffering with bipolar.

I've just come back from the Edinburgh Festival where I was playing a middle-aged lead singer of a Punk band called Sonic Generation who changed their name from Urban Castration, and my fellow cast members in the play decided I was the sanest among them. So yes, I am one of the lucky ones in that I have long spells between mood swings and now I fight everyone. That's why I am a survivor at present, and just like an alcoholic, it's one day at a time. I won't stop fighting; bipolar is going to know it has been in a battle. I know no one can fight my illness like I can and I know that ultimately it is down to me whether I continue to be a survivor or not. No matter who I look to blame, it is down to me not to give in and be another suicide.

I can fight because I have been given so much help. Help from my family, help from Dr McGowan, help from Davina Blunt and help from the inspirational Dr Jerome Carson whose friendship, understanding, laughter and recovery groups have made me realise my talents, and how much I still have to contribute to my career and to people far worse off than myself. But actually, also what I have to contribute to people generally and if I can contribute, well that's a life well lived.

Matthew Ward interviewed by Hannah Cordle

Matthew Ward's journey of recovery is a remarkable one, which has seen him come back from a suicide attempt to rebuilding his life and career as an actor. Describing his recovery as '*a work in progress*', Matthew is clear from the outset that there are more worthy people than him to be the subject of this profile. '*I feel a bit of a fraud because in under two years, with the right medication and great help, I'm charging along with a career, everything going my way, and suddenly I'm giving speeches about my recovery and recovery heroes – which is a bit too much really.*'

For Matthew, recovery is more about survival than a single defining moment when he can say he's recovered. '*I may be totally wrong and there may be people who have recovered completely, and I really hope that there are, but I don't think that will be the way for me,*' he says. '*I have been one of the lucky ones in the sense that for me recovery is being able to accept what I've got and deal with it.*'

The concept of recovery has only recently taken on meaning for Matthew. Years of mood swings and failed suicide attempts came to a head in April 2008 when he was involved in a failed theatre production, which led to a terrible low and another suicide attempt. He was picked up by the police and eventually brought to the South West Sector Community Mental Health Team in Streatham High Road. '*It had just come to a point where I was going to kill myself or I was going to get help,*' he says.

After meeting psychiatrist Dr Stephen McGowan, Matthew was prescribed lithium which worked within weeks and took the edge off the highs and lows, which in his experience of bipolar used to come at the same time and make him '*capable of anything*'. As he describes it, '*Being the life and soul of the party, buying everyone drinks in the pub, taking untold amounts of money out of my account and doing really stupid things because tomorrow I'm going to kill myself.*'

Diagnosis and medication gave Matthew the stability to begin to rationalise his illness. He says, '*Before I thought my behaviour was who I am. Now there's a reason for it and through that reason I can temper my behaviour and say "OK, that's enough".*' Matthew has also learned coping strategies which help him manage the highs and lows before they begin to engulf him. '*I've had a few highs recently where I've just stayed at home, and shut the door,*' he explains. '*When I'm on a high I'm capable of pretty much anything, so I try and avoid places where that will kick off. If I stay in one area and don't see anybody, I have more chance of coping with it than if I go out.*'

He also began attending the South West Sector Recovery Group led by consultant clinical psychologist Dr Jerome Carson. Here a diverse group of mental health service users engage with recovery through their strengths and passions, such as art, poetry and politics. These people, who Matthew describes as '*phenomenal*' became his recovery heroes by inspiring and challenging him in turn.

He says, '*Part of my recovery is that I met lots of people that were far worse off than I am, and in a strange sort of way that has really helped me because it has made me feel, OK they are dealing with it, they can cope with it,*' he says. '*With my mood swings I get huge gaps in between where I'm fine, whereas I've spoken to people in the group who are daily getting mood swings. So I felt that I'm not doing too badly.*'

A turning point came when Jerome asked Matthew if he wanted to perform a one-man play called St Nicholas for the group. '*St Nick is a tough play to do and because I knew if I couldn't do it, I wouldn't be able to go back to what I did, whether I was going to have a career or not,*' he says. That Jerome had recognised the essence of Matthew's personal identity as an actor and entrusted him to do the play was a major encouragement to Matthew. '*I could have run off, I could have done anything!*' he says. '*But I could do it because that is what I do, that is what I am.*'

This identity has needed some redefinition since Matthew has been in recovery – clearly a major task and significant achievement. '*With all employers, what I do now is tell them straightaway so there can be no comebacks afterwards,*' he says. '*So if halfway through a run I go into a mood it's because I've got bipolar. But it's never affected work.*'

A notoriously unstable profession, he describes acting as the worst profession in the world to be in with bipolar, but through Matthew's insight into his illness and his use of coping strategies, this means he doesn't have to sacrifice his belief that '*actors should really live*'. When we meet he has just returned from performing at the Edinburgh Festival. '*In Edinburgh we would finish at 12.30am and the pubs are open until 5am, there's nothing else to do, you're on a high anyway,*' he says. '*I enjoyed myself but knew that there was a cut off point. It's like another adrenaline rush on top of an adrenaline rush, and when I get that, I know it's time to go.*'

Having bipolar both helps and hinders his career. He's no longer able to learn his lines in the morning because the lithium makes him feel groggy. And because bipolar makes it difficult to concentrate he had to learn smaller chunks of dialogue for the one-man play rather than allowing one line to flow on from another. '*I do find it harder to learn my lines, but maybe it's because I've got older,*' he jokes. Despite losing the extreme highs associated with bipolar disorder, his artistic creativity remains unaffected. '*I haven't missed that as yet, it would be interesting to talk to a director who has worked with me before I was diagnosed with one who worked with me after,*' he says.

In the works of Shakespeare, Matthew has found a voice that articulates the experience of mental illness better than any other, calling Hamlet's 'To be or not to be' soliloquy '*probably the best speech ever written with regard to thoughts of suicide*'. In the same way, Matthew hopes he can give other people in recovery a voice using his acting skills, but without being a hero. '*It's very easy for me to sit here and talk about being a recovery hero but I don't think that I am,*' he says. '*I am doing all these things but I've got bipolar, and if I go and jump off a cliff next week the recovery wouldn't have worked would it?*'

Recovery is also about taking personal responsibility for your illness, according to Matthew. '*It's how much you want it, and how much you put in, is how much you'll get out,*' he says. '*I didn't really believe that before, but my mentality has changed. I'm a far more positive person than I was, in the sense that I don't think there is a golden answer that everyone will recover and everything is going to be fine. But with work and the right help and the right medication, I do think a mental illness is copeable with, for all of us.'*

An appraisal of Matthew by Jerome

What is a recovery hero? To my mind, it is someone who is battling against a major mental disorder, yet who still manages to inspire others by their deeds and actions. By these criteria, I feel Matthew scores on both counts. At a one-day recovery conference in Lambeth in May 2009, Matthew stood up to present his own story in front of over 100 professionals and service users. His presentation was entitled My Recovery: A work in progress (Ward, 2009). Matt successfully interwove his own story and battle with bipolar disorder with three verses taken from Shakespeare's Macbeth, Hamlet and King Lear. Each of these illustrated a key stage in his own life. As I sat in the audience, I felt a tremendous source of personal pride as well as admiration for this amazing actor and local service user.

Matthew mentions the play St Nicholas by the Irish playwright Conor McPherson. He put this on for our local recovery group (Morgan & Carson, 2009). Yvonne Farquharson of the Guy's and St Thomas' Charity watched his performance with us and was so impressed that she agreed to fund a short tour of this play in Lambeth. Matthew performed the play five times during an 11 day period in June 2009 and the first performance was attended by 11 people at the local YMCA. The next day he performed to 29 people at our local team base. Later that week he performed at a theatre inside the West Norwood library. This was the highlight of the first week but was again attended by a small audience of 16.

His penultimate performance was in the dining room of Lambeth Hospital where another 29 people were present. His final night was in the majestic setting of Governor's Hall at St Thomas' Hospital. There were 85 people present and I introduced each of these performances, and at the end I joined Matthew on the stage for a Q & A session about his own journey of recovery. We then asked the audience to complete a brief evaluation of the play. The results of this were very positive (Ward *et al*, 2010). Finally, we provided them all with a folder containing a number of handouts related to recovery, Matthew's own story, a copy of One in Four magazine and some information about local services. I was the only person to be present at all five performances although several of our service users went to two and one attended three performances.

In addition to the play and conference presentation, Matthew has also presented his own story at several of our recovery workshops (Carson, 2011). He also accompanied me to present to two community teams in Southwark. Along with Dolly Sen, Matthew gave an 'after dinner' speech to people completing the second set of recovery workshops that we ran for service users adding to the special nature of this event.

Matthew may be too modest to describe himself as a recovery hero. For two weeks in June 2009 and for a few weeks before this we worked intensely together to put on the five plays. I was with him for a couple of hours before each play, during the plays and after. We went through the disappointment together of only having 11 at the opening night, to the triumph of having 85 at the last night. With each performance having a Q & A session at the end, we were able to put across a positive message about recovery. Matthew believes that I have helped him with his own recovery journey. Yet, I believe he has helped and inspired many more people through his own personal witness and by showing how he has continued acting in spite of his bipolar disorder. He is to my mind a true recovery hero.

Conclusion

Matthew Ward's story illustrates how for some people getting a diagnosis can be helpful. His diagnosis of bipolar helped him see that the extreme mood swings he experienced were symptoms of an illness and not the vagaries of being an actor. We were able to use his performances of the play St Nicholas to educate people about mental illness and recovery. He has also woven in speeches from Shakespeare to help tell his own remarkable story. His acting skills have paradoxically enabled him to communicate many of the issues around recovery in a simply unique manner that has now inspired thousands of people.

References

Carson J (2011) *Recovery the long and winding road that leads*. In: H Cordle, J Fradgley, J Carson, P Holloway & Richards P (Eds) *Psychosis: Stories of recovery and hope*. London: Quay Books.

Morgan S & Carson J (2009) The Recovery Group: a service user and professional perspective. *Groupwork* **19** (1) 26–39.

Ward M (2009) *My recovery: A work in progress*. Keynote address given at Lambeth Recover Me Conference at Stockwell YMCA, May 6th (copy available from Jerome at j_carson@o2.co.uk).

Ward M, Carson J, Chander A & Robinson S (2010) It's a one man show. *Mental Health Today* 32–33.

Chapter 15

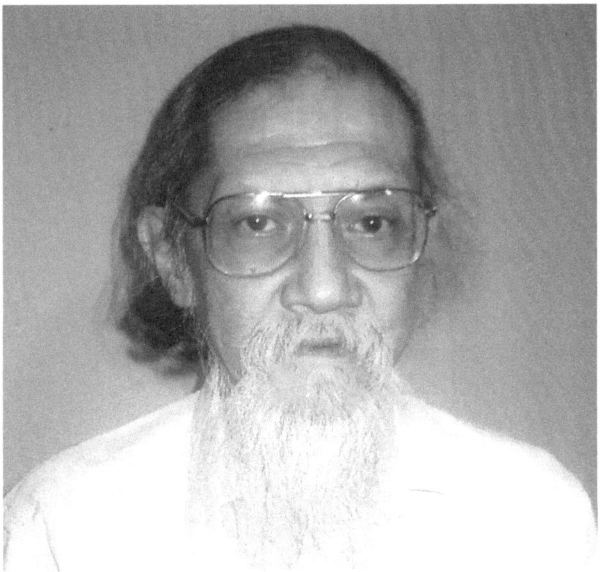

Gordon McManus

Summary

Gordon McManus set out to be a communist revolutionary. However his involvement in politics partly contributed to the development of a very serious psychotic illness, leading to four hospital admissions, and a number of 'lost years'. He was barely aware of what happened during most of the 1990s and had problems to even complete a simple form. His own natural recovery process of using writing and playing chess accelerated when his psychiatrist referred him for a course of cognitive behaviour therapy. After this, his subsequent psychological therapy led him to develop and articulate his own ideas about recovery. His definition of recovery as *'coping with your illness and having a meaningful life*' summarises the essence of the difficulties facing individuals with major mental health problems as they try to embark on their recovery journeys.

Gordon in his own words

I was born in Rangoon, Burma in 1952. I came to Britain with my parents in 1964. I attended Tulse Hill Comprehensive School from 1965 to 1970. In the 1970s, after a period of work, I attended Kingsway College of Further Education and from this institution I entered the University of Essex in 1974 where I read Linguistics with Sociology. In the 1980s, I taught Business Studies. During this period I was an active communist.

I first became ill with schizophrenia in 1991 even though I did not know it, as I was under the delusion that the Soviets were communicating with me with a new mental science. I lived with this delusion for 10 years. From 1993 to 2005, I was a '*paranoid schizophrenic*' and had five breakdowns with four hospitalisations in the process. Two of these were under a Section of the Mental Health Act. In 2001, I decided to 'rebuild' my life through writing and chess. I also resolved to repair my relationships with my family and friends.

I was under the medical model of treatment from 1994 to 2006. I was first recommended for therapy in 2006 at the Maudsley PICuP Clinic. Since 2007 I have been engaged in therapy with Dr Carson. My stage of 'recovery' begins in 2007. I am not free of 'voices' and seeing 'forms' but I am coping with them. At present I am affected with '*daily auditory hallucinations*' (in the words of Dr Carson). The nights are difficult because the voices can keep you awake all night. The usual pattern is for the voices to wake me after five to six hours sleep, between 4am and 5am. This usually lasts for about three hours. During the day I am affected by attacks of schizophrenia, but with therapy I am able to cope.

Recovery is not a cure. It is an approach to your mental health problems. Recovery for me means coping with my illness and trying to have a meaningful life. It means rationalising the illness and being aware of my problems. It means having hope and self-determination to achieve my goal of full recovery and being free of the symptoms of schizophrenia. Recovery means having good relations with family and friends, despite the illness. It means trying to 'rebuild' your personality and identifying and developing my social roles. 'Social recovery' is very important in the process of recovery. It is important to have goals no matter how small they might be. It gives me something to cling on to in the recovery journey. It means not allowing my illness to dominate me, but to try and control the effects of the symptoms, that is to say, hearing 'voices' and seeing 'forms'. The danger during the stage of recovery is having a breakdown or relapse leading to hospitalisation.

Recovery is a slow process. I feel that after four years of therapy with Dr Carson, I am halfway towards full recovery. Recovery is a struggle and involves developing one's character and showing the positive aspects of one's growth through overcoming the mental illness.

Gordon interviewed by Sarah

Gordon McManus is an ex-communist leader who still battles to control his schizophrenia. He lived a long time believing that the Soviets were controlling him. He laughs as he recounts it, but says his diagnosis '*freaked*' him out a bit. He says, '*You don't see yourself as long-term mentally ill until you get categorised that way.*'

When he first heard voices he tried to solve the problem himself. He says, '*The voices came for a few weeks.*' Then they were gone again, but were to return in two years time.

He didn't tell his family anything about his schizophrenia '*they just looked after me.*' He hid his symptoms from his doctors until one doctor said that he couldn't diagnose Gordon because he wasn't talking to him. Then Gordon said, '*I just thought I better come out and express what was happening to me. It's only now in 2009 that I can talk about recovery with some confidence. It was hard writing about my schizophrenic experiences.*' He would have liked to write more about it, but as he still hears voices he is afraid that concentrating on them may lead to another breakdown.

He calls the years that he was at his worst '*the lost years*'. He says, '*All I know is there was this form of Mugabe telling me not to use books and telephones. I feel a sense of loss for those years. The only thing that I can say that comes out during that period was some people I knew became good friends, in particular Stanton, Zimmo and Keith. We share food we share drinks. The last few years we've built a kind of relationship, which keeps me in touch with reality. They now know I suffer from schizophrenia. They didn't know during that time.'* He says that this has become a basis for making his life meaningful.

'Eric is a son of a friend of mine and in my severe period he kept me together. I broke up my friendship with him because of the voices. I only started talking to him again in 2001/02. It was a step back into making my life realistic instead of being consumed by the voices.' After coming out of hospital in 2001, Gordon resolved to rebuild his life. His illness had meant he had *'lost his intellectual function'* as he puts it.

His family has played a part in his recovery. He says, *'They show more care now* [that they know about his illness]. *In the 1990s I didn't see them that much, but since my sister became my carer in 2000/2001 they have shown an understanding of my illness.'* His younger sister gave him a computer, which he says, *'became a catalyst for change'*. He used the computer to write about politics. He says, *'it was the beginning of rebuilding myself'*. However his father died in 2002 and he broke down. He doesn't like to see this causally, *'I think I broke down because I broke down. I was quite rational about it. To this day I don't know why I broke down.'*

He says that during this time, even while he was trying to rebuild his life, *'I didn't have the concept of recovery. Never did I believe I could recover, because of two breakdowns in three years I didn't think of recovering, I just wanted to make my life more meaningful. More rational, more logical.'*

When he came out of hospital he says that he was, *'not recovered, but I could cope. I had improved.'*

Through 2005 he *'didn't do much'* as in his own words but research globalisation on the internet. He used this research on globalisation to stave off a severe bout of schizophrenia.

All of this he had done under the medical model of treatment. He had received no therapy. But in 2006 his psychiatrist decided that drugs alone were not working and referred Gordon to have therapy.

Gordon says, *'I had someone to talk to now on a fortnightly basis about my problems and it staved off hospital and breakdown.'* He says, *'I can talk about it now because I've written about it. Dr Carson has made me rationalise and objectify my illness. I had to distance myself and that came from 2005/2006, it took a long time you know.'*

Through the 1990s and up until 2001 he only had the support of the mental health system. In 2001, he told his family and one close friend about his illness. He says in 2001 the support was there.

This openness he feels is helping in his recovery, '*It means you're no longer under stress to hide things, to hide your illness. It makes it easier to keep a lot better, they understand you have your problems.*'

He says, '*I cook food for my family. I cook for friends. That's my way of giving back. It makes life a bit more meaningful. The last three or four years have been very meaningful for me.*' He says, '*I am still a paranoid schizophrenic.*' But he has learnt to manage his illness and considers himself finally as being in recovery.

He deals with the voices and 'forms' with three techniques. First, he uses chess and writing to distract himself from them. Second, is ignoring them, a technique that John Nash uses in the film *A Beautiful Mind*; the third is using the TV to distract himself.

A lot of the forms and voices that he hears are political, so the political writing helps him to deal with them. He does get more personal hallucinations and he finds those harder to deal with.

He says, '*I make that distinction between recovery and recovered. I am in recovery: coping with my illness and trying to have a meaningful life. Writing, chess and dominoes are coping techniques. I don't want to put myself under stress and break down again.*'

'*Coping means not allowing the voices to dominate you. I can't make them* [the hallucinations] *go away, that is my annoyance.*'

But he doesn't suffer from symptoms 24/7 now, or else he would be back in hospital. He has got to the point now where he can help his nephew with his school work. He says, '*Each thing is like a victory as you are still hearing voices. So that was something of a coup for me. And I didn't hear voices or see forms over it.*'

'*I try to live my life in a simple non complex way; it has to be stress free, which means the voices are not so severe. To be fully recovered that's my goal, that's what's gives me hope. That's my goal in life now. A friend of mine says to me I've come out of the dark ages. So I want this journey of recovery to be shared by others.*'

An appraisal of Gordon by Jerome

I have known Gordon for two years. I was first asked to see him by his community mental health nurse, Simon Gent. Gordon had finished a six month course of cognitive behaviour therapy (CBT) for psychosis at the Maudsley Hospital PICuP Clinic. Simon felt he would benefit from more individual work. Fortunately for me, I was the one asked to see him.

The process of recovery at an individual level is going to vary, as each individual's circumstances and life history differ. In working with Gordon, I was very impressed how he would spend weeks working on many of the papers I gave him to study (for example, Deegan, 1996: Perkins, 2006). He was always trying to relate these articles to his own experiences. I was also impressed with his developing understanding of his own recovery process. I asked him if he would present some of his ideas about recovery to our local recovery group (Morgan & Carson, 2009). The format he chose for this presentation was for me to interview him in front of the audience, and to use the model of his own recovery process as the structure of the talk (see **Figure 1** on page 149). The model shows his journey from normality, through hospital breakdown and schizophrenia, into a stage of recovery, hopefully leading back to a period of normal life.

When Gordon was ill, he felt he suffered a loss of his personality. He neglected his self-care, withdrew from social contact and communicated only with his voices. This was for him a period of irrationality. The breakthrough with his illness came in 2001. He decided to involve his family and friends more in his life. While he underwent a further episode of illness, he improved significantly after his CBT. The individual recovery work we have done together since has formed a major part of a new book we are co-editing (McManus & Carson, 2011).

It is fortunate that Gordon has been so open about his illness. He agreed to take part in the film about recovery made by Michelle McNary and his story is also told in the accompanying booklet (Carson *et al*, 2008). In addition to speaking to our recovery group, he also spoke at our recovery workshop sessions, at a local recovery conference and to a group of over 40 social work masters students. While Gordon always wanted to be known for his communist party activism and his knowledge of Marxism-Leninism, he has to my mind become better known for his reflections on recovery. When I have presented to different audiences on the nature of recovery, I always throw down a challenge of someone coming up with a more succinct

Figure 1

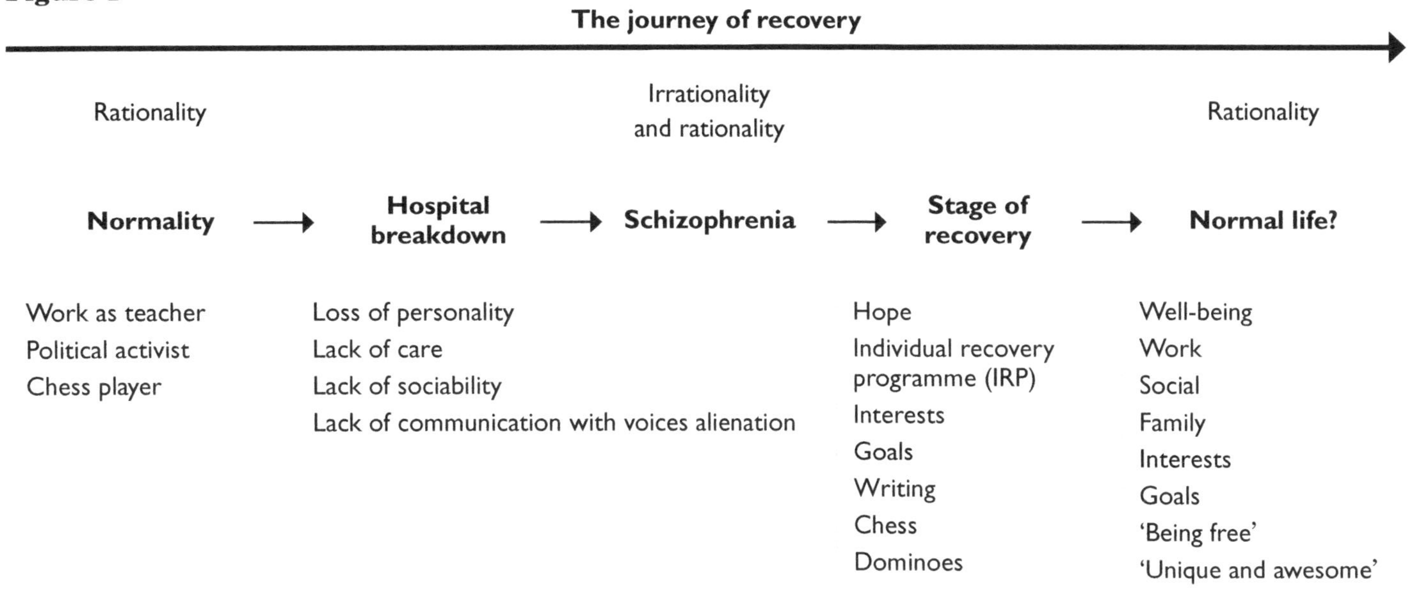

Adapted from: McManus G & Carson J (2008) One man's model of recovery. *A Life in the Day* **13** (4) 16–19.

definition of recovery than Gordon's. This is that '*recovery is coping with your illness and trying to have a meaningful life.*' Thus far, no one has been able to come up with a better definition. For so many sufferers, it can be so difficult to cope with the distressing symptoms of their mental disorders and to then also try and find a meaningful life, and not to see these years as being 'lost years'. While this of course is only one man's story, it is a story that is typical of so many sufferers. We are indebted to Gordon for sharing it and also his unique insights with us.

Conclusion

Gordon developed schizophrenia in his early 40s. He was very unwell for a number of years and was hospitalised on four occasions over a 10 year period. He worked collaboratively to develop his understanding of his condition and used his intellect to come up with a number of insights about the recovery process. He has pointed out that the two major challenges confronting everyone who is embarking on a recovery journey are how to deal with their distressing and often disabling symptoms, and how to find a life that is imbued with meaning. Neither is easy. To work in a recovery focused way may require a paradigm shift from mental health services.

References

Carson J, Holloway F, Wolfson P & McNary M (2008) *Recovery Journeys: Stories of coping with mental health problems*. London: South London and Maudsley NHS Foundation Trust.

Deegan P (1996) Recovery as a journey of the heart. *Psychiatric Rehabilitation Journal* **19** (3) 91–97.

McManus G & Carson J (2008) One man's model of recovery. *A Life in the Day* **13** (4) 16–19.

McManus G & Carson J (Eds) (2011) *From Communism to Schizophrenia and Beyond: One man's long march of recovery*. London: Whiting and Birch In press.

Morgan S & Carson J (2009) The Recovery group: a service user and professional perspective. *Groupwork* **18** (3) 26–39.

Perkins R (2006) First person 'you need hope to cope'. In: G Roberts, S Davenport, F Holloway & T Tattan (Eds) *Enabling Recovery: The principles and practice of rehabilitation psychiatry*. London: Gaskell.

Chapter 16

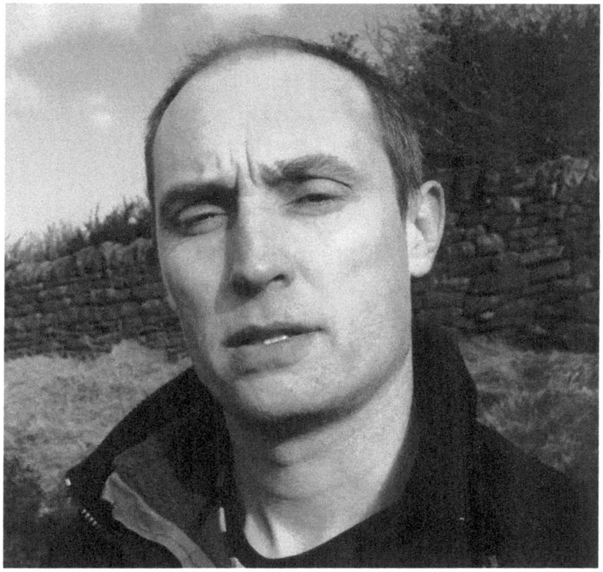

Rufus May

Summary

Rufus May is one of the best known clinical psychologists in Britain. He is known for advocating non drug-based approaches to dealing with severe mental health problems. He was admitted to psychiatric hospital on three occasions in his late teenage years and was at one time on a depot injection. Amazingly he turned his life around, stopped taking the medication and later went on to train as a clinical psychologist. He has been heavily involved in media work to dispel many of the myths surrounding psychosis.

Rufus in his own words

I think that madness is a creative way of the mind dealing with pain. We may not consciously be aware of this, but through self-understanding we can make sense of it. There are different ways to bury pain. We can invest heavily in distracting activities; we can take it out on others or take it out on ourselves. All of these strategies can lead to us becoming unstuck. My own madness was a build up of alienating experiences. I had suffered emotionally due to my mother becoming ill after a brain haemorrhage when I was eleven. I lost my way in my teenage years, investing in rebellious behaviour and avoidance of responsibility. At the age of 18 my first girlfriend left me and I found myself in a boring job with few friends. I was full of regrets and questions about my sense of belonging and purpose in the world. I was also struggling to grieve my failed relationship. To deal with these conflicts and a powerful shift in my energy, my mind chose to take me into a phantasy world. In this world, I was an apprentice British spy who was involved in a battle between East and West and good and evil. These beliefs protected me from a depressing reality and symbolised my own struggle to find values to live by and a sense of purpose in my life. I think my ideas were fuelled by buried feelings of loss triggered by the break up with my girlfriend, combined with a sense of anomie.

In mental health services no one wanted to talk to me about my experiences, instead they were cast as a biological problem called schizophrenia, which needed to be suppressed with heavy doses of stupefying psychiatric drugs. I instinctively felt that suppressing my problems indefinitely would only make me more vulnerable in the long run. I tried to come off the neuroleptic medication as soon as I was discharged from hospital. These attempts led to difficult withdrawal states, where I was hyper-energetic. These states were interpreted as relapses and confirmation that I had schizophrenia. I was put on a depot injection of Depixol. After six months, I decided to have one last attempt at stopping the medication as it was blunting me emotionally and cognitively. Doctors refused to help me with this process. I had at this stage left home and managed to find good friends to live with who were supportive. My friends were more tolerant of my chaotic behaviour, as I adjusted to not being on medication than my parents who would have been more likely to panic.

Healing happens when we can find ways to transform that buried energy that is trying to find a form of expression. I knew from my mother's rehabilitation (from her brain haemorrhage), I needed to be determined and learn new ways to express myself. I used physical exercise, drama and dance to do this. My healing and recovery also came through finding people who believed I was an equal human being with abilities and potential, and myself believing in my own self-development and recovery. There were several friends who stuck by me and believed in me, this was invaluable. Another key element was a spiritual or moral awakening that happened during my rehabilitation, where I realised to be happy, I needed to work for the benefit of others. I found when I helped others I felt good about myself, whereas if I focused solely on my own well-being, this led to me feeling isolated and lonely. I always saw my confusion not as an arbitrary affliction, but a meaningful response to life problems. I believed this was true for others too.

During my hospital admissions and journey back to independence, I saw that our society has an apartheid approach to emotional distress and confusion. There is much fear and avoidance of really listening to people suffering from confusion. This apartheid-like silence about the validity of emotional distress and the value of friendship in the healing process is rife in all social institutions, such as schools, employment and the media. I became determined to raise awareness of the need for people to be more compassionate about confusion and distressed states of mind and to think outside the medical box. I realised that I needed some social status so that people would listen to me. So I trained as a psychologist and when I had qualified and had proved myself a competent practitioner, I began to talk openly about my breakdown and recovery to help challenge negative thinking about severe mental health problems. I have over the last 12 years invested in media work, public meetings and training events to help raise awareness of holistic approaches to healing and recovery from mental health problems. Taking up a social position as an advocate for recovery for severe mental health problems has its own pressures and demands. You need to have a strong support network to push against the dominant approaches to mental health. I found it very helpful to be part of and co-create networks of like-minded thinkers, such as the Hearing Voices Network and my local Evolving Minds Network. I also use the internet to share ideas and network using my own website (see www.rufusmay.com) Facebook, YouTube and Twitter. In order to deal with the pressure I was under more effectively, I have taken up a Zen meditation practice over the last eight years which has helped me avoid being overwhelmed. Also being part of a local Quaker meeting has supported me to work creatively to promote compassionate optimistic approaches to madness and distress. Physical exercise has always helped me channel my energy more effectively and over the last few years I have taken up boxing training. Being a partner to my wife Rebecca and a father to my two boys, Gregory and Nathan, has also grounded me so that my work and activism do not totally dominate my life.

Rufus interviewed by Sophie

In his work with people with psychotic experiences, the psychologist Rufus May takes a different approach to that which he was given when he was diagnosed with '*schizophrenia*' as a young man aged 18. He believes that the medical approach to suppressing psychotic experiences by long-term use of medication does not allow someone to grow above and beyond their experiences. '*What you suppress tends to come back stronger, so it's better to address the experiences instead of just numbing them.*' Long-term medication programmes tend to cause lots of secondary health problems. It is healthier to teach people holistic strategies to calm thoughts and feelings down and find expressive activities that can channel their energy in more productive ways. Rufus is keen to make sense of people's difficulties in a collaborative way and avoids using psychiatric diagnosis.

When he was hospitalised due to his beliefs about espionage and spiritual warfare, he was told he would have to take medication for the rest of his life, '*The assumption that psychiatric diagnoses create is that someone's confusion is a lifelong condition, this can then become a self-fulfilling prophecy*'. While Rufus is critical of psychiatric diagnosis and the heavy handed use of medication he received, he acknowledges that he did '*need a place of sanctuary and some containment as well as some strategies to help him to sleep*'. This could have been through temporary use of medication but also by teaching him calming activities and encouraging physical exercise too.

Rufus believes his condition was short-lived because he had witnessed his own mother's recovery from a stroke, and he intrinsically knew the importance of determination and enabling social support. Some friends did decide not to support Rufus and he understands how this social isolation can be deeply demoralising. However other friends did not turn away from him. One particular friend visited him regularly in hospital and Rufus believes this was crucial in him not giving up on himself and the possibility of reintegrating back into society.

For Rufus, there should be tailored support for people with mental health difficulties. We need to start from the assumption that mental health problems are meaningful responses to adverse life experiences. We should be trying to collaboratively make sense of people's distress and confusion with them. Mania or depression or delusional thinking are messengers about emotional and interpersonal conflicts. We need to decode what the message is and learn from it. For Rufus there is no such thing as 'schizophrenia' because the experiences normally grouped together and defined as 'schizophrenia' differ so much from person to person and change so much over time. It may be a useful term for society and the medical profession to use to categorise people with, but in reality '*all diagnoses of schizophrenia are misdiagnoses*'.

However Rufus is not dogmatic about this. If people want to use a framework such as a diagnosis of '*schizophrenia*' to explain their mental illness he believes they should be able to, just as people are entitled to understand their lives in astrological terms if they want to. Rufus believes however that recovery is more likely if we look at the personal meanings of people's confusion, help them process their conflicts, and learn ways to calm and express emotions more productively.

Indeed Rufus' approach to dealing with mental illness is more holistic. He sees mental health crises as things that can be worked through and, crucially, as conditions which contain a meaningful message. Medication is a way of controlling that. '*If someone has a crisis and you give them medication it dampens down the symptoms, but the problem is that what you suppress comes out in different undesirable ways like lethargy*' he said. People have a choice of whether to take long-term medication or not, but in his experience of this suppression approach (which often goes hand in hand with smoking and sometimes other drug-use) people die at least 20 years earlier than they might have done if they had taken a more holistic approach.

Rufus believes that this is because mental health issues are natural. As such, dealing with them should be natural too. Therefore, if someone is panicking they should be encouraged to run on the spot or do breathing exercises and also talk about their buried feelings. In other words if someone becomes psychologically distressed or confused they should be encouraged to work that out, rather than denying its expression.

Rufus has been open about his own experiences of confusion and recovery in the media in order to promote hope and dispel myths about psychosis. He also sometimes uses his own experiences to help people on a day-to-day level in therapy sessions. He trains mental health professionals to be more open about their own personal experiences of coping with conflict as this is a valuable mutual learning tool. Rufus thinks that this use of personal experience is appreciated and leads to greater levels of trust in the therapeutic relationship. As long as we as the helper are not focusing on our own needs for consolation, sharing some level of vulnerability can make us good role models of self-awareness.

In terms of methods, Rufus uses a range of integrative approaches and is influenced by self-help networks such as the Hearing Voices Network. Through this he tries to help people to grow through empowerment, sharing coping strategies and a whole range of approaches. Holistic activities like drama, mindfulness, other non-clinical methods, such as non-violent communication and Jungian voice dialogue form a large part of his methods.

Through Jungian voice dialogue, Rufus talks to people's voices. He is one of the few people in the UK practicing such a method and is involved in training people in its use. The method does not try to get rid of the voices but rather to get people to change the relationship they have with their voices because these are part of the person's consciousness. '*I also use a lot of role play to help people practice honouring their emotions. We can use an empty chair for someone to confront an overpowering figure from their past and rehearse ways of negotiating their needs.*' Rufus also loves to use mindfulness as he believes it is a '*gentle way to help people become more compassionate to themselves and others*'. It is also a useful way for people to become more present and therefore more able to be supportive to others, he points out.

In addition, Rufus has great belief in the power of professionally assisted self-help groups. '*The group is a very powerful way to build self-acceptance and confidence*', he says. Some self-help groups he has set up have gone on to be independent self-help groups, but all hold to the values that each person has expertise and wisdom about their lives and that there is no one right way to see the world.

Rufus has been very influenced by his work with the Hearing Voices Network, which is an alliance between academics, therapists and voice hearers. It aims to promote the use of non-medical approaches such as talking therapies and self-help strategies to deal with hearing voices.

The international network founded in the late 1980s in Holland does not presume that hearing voices is an illness rather that it is one way of experiencing consciousness. Stressful voices are seen as a reaction to extremely stressful life experiences. The Hearing Voices Network aims to promote the a wider social acceptance of voice hearing and in the meantime create safe spaces where people who hear voices can get together and talk freely about their experiences.

Rufus would like cognitive behavioural therapy (CBT) to work more like the Hearing Voices Network's self-help group model. He considers CBT – used widely by the NHS and in other clinical settings – to be too expert-led a method for combating mental health problems, and has already started making links with CBT therapists to promote this idea of making CBT less formal than its current usage.

It is his belief that helping people is an art, not a science. Intuition is an essential part of helping people. '*There are some very good tools out there but you have to keep adapting them to the particular person. Society is in love with science – thinking it has all the answers*' says Rufus. He feels that psychology as a discipline has many benefits and he has learnt a lot from it and yet he also feels that it holds people back as well by trying to be objective. '*I hope psychology will learn from mindfulness and other self-help approaches which are more acknowledging of mutual wisdom and expertise and the value of self-reflection.*'

An appraisal of Rufus by Jerome

I have never met Rufus but there cannot be many clinical psychologists or mental health professionals who have not heard of him. Like me, he trained in clinical psychology at the University of East London, qualifying in 1998. In his application form, he covered up the fact that he had been diagnosed with schizophrenia and had been hospitalised three times. He reasoned that if the clinical training courses knew his history of mental illness, he would not have been accepted to do his clinical training. He was almost certainly correct in this assumption. Once he was clinically qualified and working in his first job, he 'came out' about his history of psychosis (May, 2000).

Rufus is probably best known for being the psychologist featured in the Channel Four documentary, *The Doctor Who Hears Voices* made by the director Leo Regan. In this, Rufus is seen treating a young doctor (played by an actress) who suffered with hallucinations, without the doctor taking medication for her symptoms. Rufus showed how to treat her condition using only a psychological approach. The programme not surprisingly generated a lot of controversy.

In addition, and to the best of my knowledge, Rufus is the only clinical psychologist featured in Wikipedia. His entry is summarised thus:

'Rufus May is a British clinical psychologist best known for using his own experience of being a psychiatric patient to promote alternative recovery approaches for those experiencing psychotic symptoms. After formally qualifying as a clinical psychologist, he then disclosed that he had previously been detained in hospital with a diagnosis of schizophrenia.'

Rufus was interviewed by Fergal Keane for the Radio Four programme Taking a Stand (see www.rufusmay.com for a full transcript of the interview). In this revealing interview he discloses how he came close to death on one occasion:

'I just started walking down the track and the train came up behind me and I heard the hooter and I froze and it just stopped in front of me, just beside me, and I got onto the train and I was preoccupied with religious ideas at the time and I said, "Do you believe in Jesus?" The train driver said, "I don't know about him, but it's a good job Harry saw you!"'

A good job indeed.

Conclusion

There are striking parallels between the story of Rufus and that of Patricia Deegan and Emma Harding. All three individuals developed a psychotic illness before later going on to train as clinical psychologists. Rufus has been very active in the media, using his own experiences of the psychiatric system to draw attention to the flaws in the system. He has also been very involved in helping develop service users' networks, and in establishing mutual self-help. His own recovery story can be a beacon of hope for many sufferers.

References

May R (2000) Roots to recovery from psychosis: the roots of a clinical psychologist. *Clinical Psychology Forum* **146** 6–10.

Chapter 17

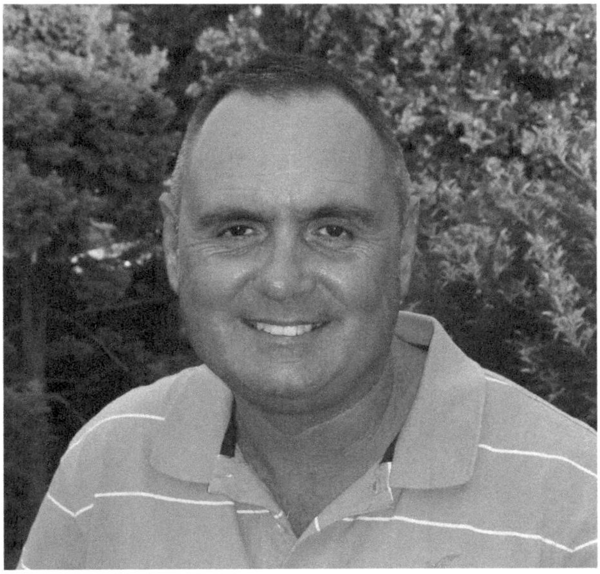

Peter Bullimore

Summary

Peter Bullimore was sexually abused as a child by the family babysitter. This led to him hearing voices. These problems resurfaced when he had a breakdown later in life that led him to be sectioned several times. He was in danger of becoming a chronic psychiatric patient. Meeting an occupational therapist who believed in him and attending a Hearing Voices Group helped transform his life. Miraculously he made a dramatic personal recovery, although he still hears voices. He has traveled all over Britain and overseas to tell his story, helping hundreds of service users both cope and learn to live with their voices.

Peter in his own words

I feel that having told my narrative many times it was about time to fill in some of the gaps as it is not possible to put eight years of abuse and 10 years in the system into a few pages. I hope this will highlight the arduous journey that I have taken but also inspire others to reclaim their lives. I remember all too well the incidents that on reflection people must have noticed, but I didn't. I was running a business that gave me wealth and a lifestyle that I had only ever dreamed of but as time went on it became my enemy and started to destroy my soul. I had become obsessed with money and power and didn't care who I hurt to achieve it: this was a stark contradiction of my working class values. I began to realise that I was controlled by the business and there was no way out, the feeling of powerlessness at times would overwhelm me, bringing back the painful memories of child abuse when I was powerless. I felt that the only way out was to self-destruct. I decided I was going on my journey to destruction before my whole existence imploded. I would finish work around 10.30pm and head for the pub most nights. By 11.30pm, I would have drunk five pints of beer and five large whiskies – surely the police would stop me and arrest me and help me out of what was now becoming a nightmare. I could not believe it, I never got stopped. I started to believe that the world was conspiring against me again just like when no one saved me from being abused as a child. My paranoia was now raging. I felt like my life was built out of playing cards and with one push, it would all be over. Why wouldn't anyone push hard enough? Why was I being punished?

The Sunday, the day of my outer body experience, it was my father's birthday. We went to the local pub in the afternoon. I was drinking crazily. My father sensed something was wrong but I couldn't get drunk enough to escape the life I hated. Was the landlord giving me weak beer? Was he in the plot to punish me? Had the world turned against me because of what I had become? I wanted the day of reckoning to come to put me out of my misery. That evening I had an outer body experience and my descent into full-blown madness had begun.

During my madness I have recalled many humorous moments, some of which will be highlighted in the book I hope to write later. One that sticks in my mind was when I believed I was receiving messages from God. These messages would be passed to me through the letters on car registration plates. I saw one with the letters BWG. I was sure this meant Big White God. The next car was AWF. This I believed stood for A World

Famine. Therefore, God had chosen me to save the world from a famine. I decided that when all the food was gone, I would save everyone by growing turnips. I spent days going around shops buying turnip seeds. I had hundreds upon hundreds of packets. This was my chance of redemption. Unfortunately for me this became an obsession. I would be going into clothes shops, newsagents, any shop I found, and I would demand them to sell me the seeds. As you can imagine this soon got back to services and once again hospital beckoned. The curious thing was when I returned home from hospital all the seeds had gone and no one would ever admit to taking them. I hope this gives you an overview. I hope one day to sit down and put the whole story together and take the reader onto a journey of sadness, madness, laughter, but most of all give them hope. On reflection I wouldn't change one day of my life. It made me who I am and I can confidently say I like myself again.

Peter interviewed by Sophie

Peter was sexually abused from the age of eight. At this time the voices were very comforting and they went on for quite some years. But then they took a very destructive turn and he started to think unpleasant thoughts about breaking his own limbs or trying to make himself sick on toothpaste. This continued in the same vein until he was aged about 13.

When the abuse finally stopped the voices went away but on becoming a parent, Peter found that the voices returned, partly because he developed a fear that something terrible would happen to his own children. This began when his first son was born – he was simply overcome by a massive sense of fear. In the early 80s, circumstances became more even more unstable when Peter became involved in organised crime.

He started working seven days a week and thought of himself as a 'big time gangster' in his own words, and yet he never told his wife about the voices. Soon he was working 18-hour days, seven days a week and the pressure built up. He would still be out at work at midnight and he would find it very hard when his wife rang up and criticised him for it. Instead of letting on about the reality of the situation, Peter would disassociate himself from what she was saying and start to think that she was trying to tell him something else. He ended up getting extremely paranoid, and thinking that the world was out to get him. He would drive three hours out of his way if he knew someone was coming over so he didn't have to see them.

On one particularly bizarre occasion, his wife invited a social worker to come and visit him and Peter walked into the room to hear lots of voices. He took one look at the social worker and was convinced she was a French spy, even though she was in fact an old lady.

It got to the point where he was also experiencing very bad insomnia and going to see the GP was the only option. He even had an out of body experience in which he thought he'd died. He simply wasn't recovering. By this point, Peter had become a 'real wreck' in his own words. He resorted to going to see the psychiatric services and was duly put on medication.

In just two months he had gone from being a working man to a psychiatric patient. He found he could no longer control his actions. He would, for instance, leave work at midnight and go to the pub where he would have five large whiskeys and five pints of beer. He used to think a character from the film *Nightmare on Elm Stree*t was lurking in the back of his van.

By this stage he was on medication but had not been formally diagnosed. A psychiatrist now told him, '*Mr Bullimore, you're a chronic schizophrenic – go away and live your life*.' He was having terrifying nightmares around this time. Once he woke up screaming to find that he couldn't see his wife who was trying to comfort him. He tried to strangle her but she managed to push him off. This signalled Peter's first sectioning. He was aged 28.

Nothing was improving and he tried suicide. It was, Peter now believes, very fortunate that his therapist never asked him his diagnosis. He felt like she understood him and didn't judge him. Peter also believes he had a very good psychiatrist. By this stage he wasn't washing and wasn't talking coherently. On the advice of a social worker, he went along to a hearing voices group in Sheffield. He listened to people talking about their lives and thought that this is where he belonged.

People were well-dressed and talked about their recovery. They related the voices to what was happening in their lives. Then a very clever guy at the Hearing Voices Group said, '*Peter, just because you hear voices doesn't mean you're mad.*' This was a revelation. He stopped going to the group and stopped seeing Sally, his therapist, thinking he could do it on his own.

Peter had been used to employing nine people on the shop floor. He had started to think they were his disciples and that he had died and been resurrected. In retrospect he can see that this was actually quite logical.

One time he went into Sheffield Cathedral and thought that he should have been having the Last Supper. He jumped into the pulpit and the vicar, in shock, shouted, '*Christ Almighty!*' Peter's response, thinking he was Christ, was naturally, '*Brilliant – I've been recognised at last!*'

In his worsening condition, Peter started to think that maybe he had been born to kill himself. But when he went to see Paul his psychiatrist, he couldn't remember the word for 'myself' so he ended up telling him that he thought he was born to kill. As a result Peter got sectioned and the psychiatrist moved to another trust out of fear.

In Peter's view, it is always necessary for mental health practitioners to ask the simple yet very necessary question of '*what actually happened to service users to make them like they are.*' He was asked for rectal examinations, for instance, which naturally made him uncomfortable, given his history of sexual abuse. Equally he would sometimes feel uncomfortable around female therapists who were talking loudly. None of this would have made any sense to anyone unless they asked why he was uncomfortable, and what had actually happened to him.

Peter's mother dying was a real turning point. There were 200 people at the funeral, but Peter never cried. He thought he would die if he cried. Shortly after he doused himself in petrol, set himself on fire and walked into a day centre. As a consequence he was sectioned again, but Sally his therapist wouldn't let him slip through the net. The divorce came through but he still had three children to care for, which helped.

Peter managed to refind the Hearing Voices Group and was invited to Sheffield to do a workshop. The same studious guy, who had given him good advice before, now said that he needed to address the demons of his past. So Peter came to realise that the only power that his abuser still had was in fact what he was letting her have. He told himself that she couldn't do anything to him anymore. He started to listen intently to the voices and realised that the worst ones were his abuser. He also started to realise that he hadn't dealt with the abuse. The abuse was not his fault – he had not chosen it – and yet despite looking the abuser in the eye he had not looked the emotional side of his abuse in the eye.

He felt an enormous amount of guilt about the abuse and the pleasure it had given him. Abuse is always multi-layered, Peter thinks. So he decided to literally put himself on trial, creating a pretend court of law in his head.

He was afraid that he would find himself guilty but then realised that in the past he had been urinated on in a stairwell, he had lost everything – it didn't matter if he found himself guilty. In listening to the voices he realised how demonic they were. He had let the abuser dominate and get away with it. He decided he was going to challenge her, and the recovery was very rapid after that.

Peter says he is still quite similar now. He still hears the voices and is still a workaholic, which he always has been. If he overworks too much, the voices start to go crazy and get totally out of hand. Peter realised that when he was a child, the voices would begin when he was feeling vulnerable. He now knows that the voices come as an early warning signal that he is feeling vulnerable again. He doesn't think he'll ever fully recover but looks at it as a positive thing now as it's a part of him.

He always has the fear that the voices will become overwhelming again, but now he has a way of controlling them. The springtime is always the hardest time of year because his parents and his son all died around that time, so he has to constantly fight the voices and not let them get on top of him.

An appraisal of Peter by Jerome

I remember reading Peter's account of his upbringing and his contact with psychiatric services when Hannah Cordle had interviewed him for P*sychosis Stories of Recovery and Hope* (Bullimore, 2011). I thought then what a remarkable man he must be. I subsequently got to meet him briefly at the Mind Media Awards as he had been doing some work with the BBC World Service. After this, I persuaded him to come to London to speak to our local recovery group, which he did in December 2010. Like Augusto D Mello (see Chapter 19), Peter is a very charismatic speaker. He was chosen to speak at the Health Talk Online launch of their page on psychosis (see 'schizophrenia' in their list of conditions at www.healthtalkonline.org). Peter is featured in two video clips as are Stuart Baker-Brown and Dolly Sen.

When Peter came to our Streatham team base there were 16 people there to hear him. He spent a total of eight hours travelling there and back to speak to us and could only stay for an hour. Peter took us through his individual story, which virtually mirrored the account in our book. I got the sense that he knew his own story by heart and that he had probably given that talk hundreds of times. His observations on the psychiatric system were both perceptive and telling. He talked of staff using expressions about patients like, '*That person's lights went out years ago.*' Comments such as this are of course profoundly damaging. Sitting there listening to Peter talk, I felt disappointed that more people were not present to hear this amazing man. He is a very inspiring and motivating speaker. Peter used no visual aids but was able to help us conjure up images simply by his powers of description. He is undoubtedly one of the most impassioned and impressive speakers I have ever heard in the mental health field. You can see him yourself on the Health Talk Online and on the BBC World Service website. In his Health Talk Online interview, he has this to say about recovery:

'To be honest, I don't get that involved ... in recovery, because I think it's wrong why we are telling people how to recover ... Man has recovered from all sorts of things since he walked this planet ... what he needs is love, compassion and guidance, we don't need tools for recovery, we don't need models for recovery ... we're turning recovery into a science it has been hijacked by the services ...'

Whose recovery is it anyway? It is of course the service users' recovery (Social Perspectives Network, 2007). As Peter says, let us make sure that mental health professionals do not steal it!

Conclusion

Peter Bullimore went from having a successful business making fireplaces to being a chronic mental patient after experiencing a serious schizophrenic breakdown. Several admissions followed his first and he seemed destined to become a 'revolving door' patient. Amazingly, he was able to break this cycle through working with a few staff who believed in him, and also through his contacts with the Hearing Voices Network. He now works as a mental health trainer both nationally and internationally.

References

Bullimore P (2011) Forging his own destiny. In: H Cordle, J Fradgley, J Carson, F Holloway & Richards P (Eds) *Psychosis Stories of Recovery and Hope*. London: Quay Books.

Social Perspectives Network (2007) *Whose Recovery is it Anyway?* London: Social Perspectives Network.

Chapter 18

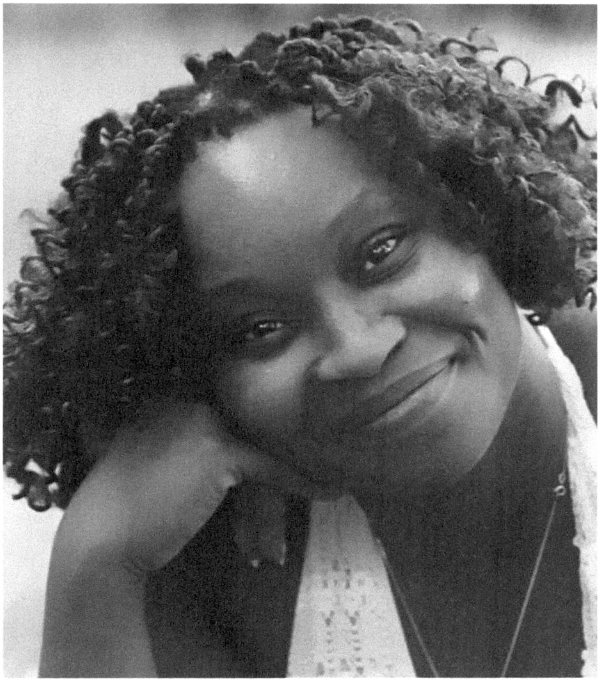

Bose Dania

Summary

Bose describes how her interest in performing arts led to her travelling to Austria to take part in a show. She stayed on to teach but had a major breakdown and was admitted to hospital in Austria. This was the start of a long period of admissions to psychiatric units in England. Her condition has now stabilised with hard work from Bose and the support of her partner and family. Her struggles are expressed in the poetry that she has written through these periods.

Bose in her own words

I was born in Lagos, Nigeria, while my mother was visiting family there, but I consider myself to be a Londoner. I remember my childhood as being very difficult. My parents separated when I was six months old; at one stage, my mother, my stepdad and six of us children lived in a two bedroom flat. School was also tough as I had dyslexia although this wasn't diagnosed until I was 32.

My childhood dream was to perform and become like Michael Jackson, my idol. I studied Performing Arts at Westminster Kingsway College but due to my dyslexia I didn't do well in my written work. I wasn't put off and tried again later enrolling in a BTech course at Barking College, which I helped pay for by working as an usherette at the Theatre Royal in Stratford. I finished college at 19 and decided to put on a show that I called Black, Proud and Beautiful, which I wrote, directed and choreographed myself.

My big breakthrough was getting a three month job playing Porgy and Bess in Austria, and I fell in love with the natural beauty of Austria. Fortunately, I was asked if I would be interested in teaching some dance classes there, but to get some more money I needed to take on some additional teaching commitments. While I was allowed to rent a hall free of charge, it proved difficult to recruit students. I decided to do my own PR and I contacted the TV and the local newspapers. This did the trick and soon I was running dance classes every day of the week and at weekends, I was a 'freestylist' when visiting pop stars were in town.

The combination of hard work and partying took its toll. I did not speak German and this led to feelings of paranoia that people might be talking about me. I decided I better try and escape back to London. However, inexplicably I spent an entire day trudging between the railway station and the dance studio, until eventually I was picked up by the local police. I was taken down to the station where they arranged for me to see a doctor. The outcome of this was that I was taken by ambulance to a mental hospital, and there, I was put on medication. The only way I could get discharged was by asking my family to come over to Austria to take me home.

On my return to London I volunteered to help with a women's health project just to keep myself occupied. I then had another psychotic episode. This time I believed there was a bomb in my room and if I moved it, it would explode. At the time I was living in a bed and breakfast place. I decided I ought to tell the other residents there was a bomb. Someone decided to call an ambulance and I found myself in another psychiatric hospital. This was one of seven admissions I was to have over a three year period. One big lesson I learned was that deterioration in my mental health was linked to smoking weed, which prior to this I had done regularly. When I stopped smoking my partner said he saw a big improvement in me.

The help I have had from services has varied over the years. One particular psychiatrist was very good to me and while he was a very busy man, he always seemed to find some time for me in his schedule. For me, volunteering was one of the key elements in my own recovery. At one stage, I worked for five days a week in a charity shop in Lewisham and I also did some work for the Afriya Trust (the Afriya Trust is a national charity that works to reduce inequalities in health and social care provision for people from racialised communities).

Really the people who have helped me the most have been my family, my partner and also my son. When I was in hospital I missed my son and this gave me the motivation to get better. Likewise, it meant a great deal when my partner came to visit me.

Writing poetry has been very therapeutic for me. I wrote my first poetry book, *A Silent Cry*, when I was at college, and later followed my next book, *Guidance of Time*.

I recently gave a talk at a psychosis conference in London in front of 250 people, which was very nerve wracking for me. Luckily, a friend came with me for support and I persuaded Jerome to let me sell some of my poetry books on the day. I ended up selling over 100 copies. I'd really like to develop my poetry more and give performances of my poetry to different groups; that of course and looking after my son.

Bose interviewed by Sophie

Bose Dania used to be professional dancer. After training in London she went out to Austria to dance as well as train dancers and finally ended up running her own successful dance school. When the signs of psychosis started to appear she simply kept on working. She didn't know anything about mental illness and never thought she could fall prey to it. She didn't want to admit that she might have a problem or, even worse, needed help.

Bose had five episodes before she was given a diagnosis of bipolar illness. In order to get out of the hospital her family had to come and get her and take her back to London. Two weeks later she returned to Austria but then it dawned on her that something was not right. She was forced to come back to London permanently in May of the year 2000 having spent three years in Austria.

For Bose, it was very hard letting go – she had a lovely apartment and a great job, so for her the loss of everything was terrible. '*I just wanted to die*' she commented. Recovery, she admits, was a very long journey. In three years she had a total of seven episodes.

She spent around a year and a half in self-confessed self-pity, even going back to Austria four times and saying goodbye to it each time. When she finally realised there was nothing in Austria to go back for she started to get her confidence back.

Her family was crucial to her recovery, giving her a lot of support and reminding her of the many things she had achieved, like starting a business in a country where she didn't even speak the language. She also started to make TV and radio appearances which served to remind her of all that she had achieved.

In fact getting the diagnosis made things easier because she was now able to differentiate better between when her character was taken over by the illness and when she was being herself. If she was having a bad day she could now put it down to the illness rather than feeling bad about herself, so she'd give herself a break, sit on the sofa and watch television and think '*tomorrow is a different day*'.

Bose also took on volunteer work which gave her back a routine. She volunteered for Cancer Research, among other activities; she also started working with mental health groups. In a process of general empowerment, she started to learn about her rights and what was and wasn't right for her with different types of medication.

All this gave her a sense of personal initiative and was really important in the process of self-understanding and recovery. She also did some work for City and Hackney Mind, including writing a newsletter which she started from scratch. She wrote an article for them about the experience of giving up smoking weed, something she also believes aided her recovery.

Slowly but surely Bose's confidence was being rebuilt as she started to get involved in more and more work in mental health. Now she began partaking in everyday pleasurable activities again like going on holiday, visiting friends and writing. '*I was basically finding myself again*' she commented.

Bose also met her partner in 2006 and had a son a year later in November 2007, both of which were real turning points. When she had her son she came off the medication for a year and a half, but then had a relapse when her son was three months old. It was Bose's first relapse in four years and the diagnosis then changed from bipolar to schizoaffective disorder.

Bose's son has been a real inspiration to her, and another reason to try and prevent any further relapse. She doesn't want him to grow up with memories of her in hospital. As he was only three months old when she had an episode, she knows that he can't remember it but is aware that if she were to have an episode now, he most definitely would.

Writing has also become increasingly important to her and become a further means of aiding her recovery. Bose had enjoyed writing before the illness and she took it up again when she had regained enough strength. She regularly writes poetry and has published several poetry books, which she sells at poetry performances. The most recent is called, *Life After Diagnosis*. She has her own website, which tells people about her story and her recovery. She talks and presents her work at all sorts of events.

In addition, Bose has been engaged in writing a book about recovery called *Understanding the Journey* since 2003. Through the book, she hopes to inspire others to find themselves again after mental illness. She wants people to know that it really is possible to get through it. She has so far written 70 pages and is looking forward to finishing it soon. In it, she tries to describe the experience of having psychotic episodes so that others can understand better the experience of having a mental illness. As with everything, her partner has been a real support with the book. As Bose is dyslexic, he checks what she has written for accuracy of spelling.

Bose had to really fight her demons to enable her recovery. There was a lot of emotion that she needed to deal with. Before the illness, she was always very busy. When she had time off she smoked weed, drank and basically pretended everything was okay. In order to get better, therefore, she had to face her family and talk about some issues that needed talking about which had been avoided for years. When she met her partner he taught her that it's okay to express emotions. She used to think that a person shouldn't cry as it is a sign of weakness.

'The process of recovery is a really long process – so long it's hard to explain,' she said. *'You've got to really want it to beat it. I don't go to church but I do believe that things happen for a reason, even if you don't necessarily know the reason at the time. Before the illness I was a real "power person" but now I am more rounded. I might not have met my partner before the illness, or if I had I might not have realised how wonderful he is,'* she said.

You also need a reason for wanting to get better, whether it be your children, your partner, your work, or simply because you want to get better, says Bose. None of her friends have mental illness, and she likes it that way because she finds that having friends with mental illness and talking to them about it can drag her as well as them down. All her friends are busy, they go to work, they have full daily routines. She is happy about that because she finds them to be inspiring.

An appraisal of Bose by Jerome

Bose was another of the people that Hannah Cordle interviewed for our book on psychosis (Dania, 2011a). Hannah was very enthused by her meeting with Bose, who as her story illustrates had a prolonged period of mental illness with multiple admissions. Unusually for a book we were given a grant by the Guy's and St Thomas' charity to write the book on psychosis. Each person was given £100 for their contribution and due to NHS bureaucracy, this money was paid out very slowly and Bose's tenacity in chasing up this payment meant that our office manager paid her separately. It was a similar tenacity that led her to negotiate a fee from me for the conference and the opportunity to be able to sell her poetry books. She has learned from experience that if you don't ask, you don't get!

In 32 years of working in mental health services, one of the most positive changes has been the emergence on an independent service user voice. In Bose's case, she is telling her own story through her poetry (see www.daniaspoetrycorner.co.uk). I have only met her in person once, but once met, she is never forgotten – such is the infectious warmth of her personality. It seems fitting to end with one of her poems entitled *Thank You*, which in her book, *Life After Diagnosis*, she dedicates it *'to all the nice nurses and social workers, that I have met along the way.'*

Thank You

You try to care
In a system of red tape
And paper work
That makes it easy
To switch off and just meet
The government's criteria
But you somehow find a way
To show you care and even when
You don't understand
You show love and compassion
Becoming a friend and not just
A nurse or a social worker
For through the red tape and paper work
You take time to see the person
Behind the illness
Far and few you may be
But still you are appreciated
So to you I say
Thank you for your kindness

(Dania, 2011b)

Conclusion

Bose had always been interested in performing arts. She travelled to Austria to take part in a show and then stayed on to open up her own dance school. After a period of overwork, she had a breakdown and her family had to bring her back to England. In a period of three years she had a further seven admissions. In addition to her interest in dance, she has always loved writing poetry and she has written several short poetry books. Settling in a relationship and having her son have given her much more stability in her life and she is now more optimistic about her future than she has been for several years.

Reference

Dania B (2011a) *Bold, Black and Beautiful*. In: H Cordle, J Fradgley, J Carson, F Holloway & Richards P (Eds) *Psychosis Stories of Recovery and Hope*. London: Quay Books.

Dania B (2011b) *Life After Diagnosis* [online]. Available at: www.daniaspoetrycorner.co.uk (accessed July 2011).

Chapter 19

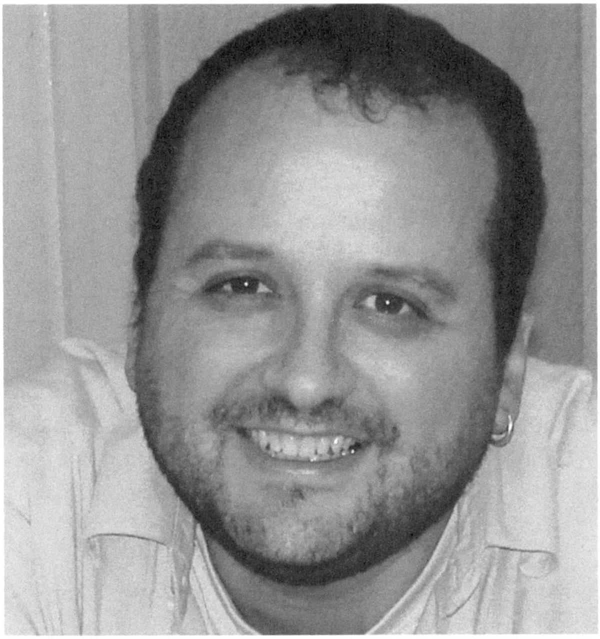

Augusto D Mello

Summary

Augusto talks about the importance of recognising the talents that each individual possesses and not being held back by illness. His breakdowns could be seen as breakthroughs: the solution is to try and work towards happy and fulfilling lives by embracing our uniqueness. He has developed a wellness toolbox to promote well-being.

Augusto in his own words

'My arms are down, my heart is open. I am naked in a land of warriors'.

What is it we want? The one thing we all desire? As John Lennon wrote, and I agree, '*all we need is love*'. More specifically, we all want to give and receive love – even the least passionate person strives for a loving relationship.

Some of us establish such a relationship with one another, others with their pets, even with a car, a house or a garden. I see nothing wrong with it.

However, for a reason that defies my comprehension, I was taught from an early age that I had to be careful about opening up too much, that society was 'cold and cruel'. I started believing sensitivity was a sign of weakness. I had to always keep my head up and '*fight*' to achieve my goals – so I did, I put on my emotional armour and left ready for battle – and I was not alone.

And here comes the contradiction – because so many of us leave our house every morning emotionally protected and with our hearts closed, our worst nightmare of not being able to love or being loved becomes a reality, and more, we end up indeed in a distant and cold society as a whole.

This is the insight I had from my first 'break through' 15 years ago as my dear friend, George Wood, calls it. And it came with an amazing emotion – for a week I was touched with this intense feeling. If I were to use a word to describe it that would be '*agape*' – transcendental love – although agape describes only an infinitesimal part of what I felt.

As I tried to talk about it to others, I saw many stupefied faces but not one that I could connect with or truly share what I was going through. I was emotionally naked; and it felt so lonely.

As time went by I never lost touch with that amazing feeling, even as I had to overcome many challenges in the years that followed; including a diagnosis of bipolar affective disorder two years later, 10 hospital admissions (9 times of which I was sectioned against my will) within 9 years and with many losses.

There were two things that kept me going, firstly I knew that at least that first experience was real and no one or anything could take that away from me; and secondly, a commitment – if I had to fall 1,000 times, a 1,000 times I would rise up again and keep pushing the boundaries.

Now, I finally learnt how to manage this unique little light of mine, which I desire so much to let shine as bright as it can be.

I was once inspired by a great care manager and today I believe that the solution for us who or have had unusual experiences commonly labelled with a mental health diagnosis, is to achieve happy and fulfilling lives. Rather than try to 'squeeze' ourselves into the box of the majority, we can grow and thrive in a slightly bigger box. As Patricia Deegan (1996) has said, instead of being forced to join the mainstream of society, we need the stream to become wider, so we can all be included.

There is nothing wrong in having unusual experiences as long as we are on 'top of them' – they don't cause suffering to ourselves or others. This is a balance that is not easy to be achieved, but it is definitely worth it.

There is so much we can contribute to our society as we are without the need to be put back 'into line' by being stuffed up with excess medication. Please, don't get me wrong, I believe it is important for me to take as much meds as necessary to keep me in the right side of the 'borderline', but not far from it. I want to be close enough to keep gently pushing it, always.

Augusto interviewed by Sophie

For Augusto, the stigma attached to the words 'mental health' comes from associations with aggressive behaviour mainly disseminated by mainstream media, therefore whenever anyone asks what he does, he answers that he works in the field of '*promoting healthy minds*'. He finds this a far more positive and empowering way of getting the message across. He believes in the power of the word 'mind' because, in his own words, '*Mind transcends brain – brain is just a machine – and though it is a brilliant machine, it is also limited to automated responses to stimulus, our mind, on the other hand, holds a much more abstract level of being which encompasses our very self.*'

Augusto has been working as a consultant and trainer with professionals and clients in this field for over four years. Diagnosed with bipolar affective disorder 13 years ago, Augusto believes he has recovered and is now able to manage what he calls vulnerability rather than illness, and what he considers to be part of his makeup as a unique human being.

'*For nine years the best I could do was to keep my head above water, it took me a long time to realise I could learn how to swim!*' he comments. '*If there is a word to define my experiences in that period, I believe the best word is loss – I lost friends, work and my own identity. My relationship with my wife was heavily affected, even the way I related to my parents changed. They were still very loving, but became much more cautious in the way they approached me.*'

Augusto hasn't had a major crisis for over five years now. He is evidently delighted.

His main tool for self-managing has been what he calls '*the power of slow*'. As soon as he realises he is losing his balance, he starts moving much slower than his usual pace, '*Even if it is just my fingers, I move them very slowly. I realised that just by slowing down my body movements, I send a powerful message to my brain which reacts to it and soon I regain control and I am back to the place I like to be*'.

He uses this simple technique whenever he needs it. He does not like to compare it to a meditation because of its usual connection to religion and the fact that, although often denied, usually there is a philosophy attached to it, he explains. '*The power of slow is very simple and as soon as you attach a philosophy to it you lose it*', he adds. '*It works amazingly well, I even call it my "golden tool" because it is also effective when I am starting to feel low – as I slowly accomplish things rather than giving in to depression. I naturally feel better. It is my most valued tool because it is so simple, easy to do and effective.*'

'*Another great recovery tool is simply joy. The ability to feel joy is one of the first things to disappear when depression tries to creep in.*' According to Augusto, supporting someone in finding things that can provide them with joy, even small glimpses of it – whatever that may be – is one of the most effective ways of helping them out of their suffering. '*Better yet is to combine both tools! For example, I love mocha coffee, hence if I realise I am starting to get either high or low, whenever I can, I go to a lovely coffee shop and very slowly enjoy an extra large cup. For me, it works wonders,*' he says.

Augusto agrees that recovery is a journey; however he finds the idea that it is an *'on-going process'* disempowering and demotivating since for him it implies that one is always ill because one is always recovering. He believes that when the process of recovery starts, so does the management process of one's condition. Recovery, in his opinion, can and does happen and only the person going through it can pinpoint when it does. *'When we recover, what is left is a higher vulnerability than most people have, but which in my opinion is not an illness – it is an aspect of who we are – managing that is on-going.'*

Augusto also believes recovery has many aspects and therefore many *'different journeys'*. He says, *'I feel I recovered from being ill; I am, however, still recovering from some of the effects which that period had in my life.'* He is still working on his personal relationships, for example, *'The support of my wife, Tania and loved ones has been key to my life, but there is much recovery and healing still to be done in that area, and I am not sure how long that journey will take, and in this journey, I am not travelling by myself.'*

Nonetheless in many aspects of his life he is in fact managing successfully: he stopped receiving incapacity benefit and has built a new career, which he really enjoys, and he has earned much respect and is considered to be one of the best service user presenters around today.

He knows that if he has a relapse he will have to undergo the journey of recovery once again, he says, *'And I know it would never be an easy process, but I also know it can be achieved and no one or anything can take that away from me. Also, with each recovery process I go through, I learn more about myself, life, and what has real value and matters most to me.'*

According to Augusto, many people who have similar experiences adopt the idea that being diagnosed with a mental illness is a kind of *'life sentence'* and they end up losing hope and getting stuck. *'That is heart-breaking,'* he says.

Augusto is also realistic about recovery. He knows that one cannot go back to being the person they were before the illness. *'Many people want to be the person that they were before, but of course the clock can't turn backwards. We can't even be the person we were yesterday. The essence of life is that things change and after such traumatic experiences we just can't see or feel the world as if nothing happened. The way forward is to let go and ask ourselves the big questions: who am I now? And then what is it I want to accomplish from where I stand today?'*

For Augusto, the choices made at this stage are crucial. '*It is imperative that one regains the power to make his/her own choices no matter how challenging it is to let go of the past*', he says. '*We build our sense of self of who we are and what reality is since the moment we are born; it is no surprise how incredibly unsettling it feels when we lose them all.*'

Augusto was inspired by an observation of Tony Walford, his care manager, who once said to him that everybody sometimes feels enthusiastic or happy, sad or angry, but that in Augusto's case his range of emotions is wider than that of most people. Tony also said he was not there to squeeze him into the box of the majority, but to make sure he was safe. This simple observation was life changing for Augusto, as he had never looked at it that way before. He realised that there was nothing wrong in being slightly different than the majority, as a matter of fact; he could flourish as he was, also making sure, himself, that he was safe.

And to be safe he believes there is no better '*medication*' than self-knowledge, '*It's said that in the oracle of Apollo, in Greece, it was written in bold letters "know thyself". For most people, the journey of self-knowledge is a luxury, for us who have been touched by such powerful experiences it is a must. Only through profound understanding of who we are and, more importantly, who we want to be, we can steer our life in the direction we want and have the best possible chance to get there.*'

An appraisal of Augusto by Jerome

My first encounter with Augusto was when I was chair of a morning session, on the third day of the refocus on recovery conference. He was the 'lived experience' speaker for that session and I was to introduce him to the audience and ensure that he kept to his allocated time. The venue for this presentation was the main lecture theatre of the Friends Meeting House near Euston Station in London. There were over 300 delegates present when Augusto got up to talk. In his interview with Sophie, she points out that he has been '*considered to be one of the best service user presenters around today*' and indeed I was so impressed personally with him that morning that I invited him to give a keynote address at our psychosis conference. He did not disappoint that day either. Augusto is a very charismatic speaker.

One of the main foci of Augusto's work is an emphasis on well-being. This is of course very popular at the moment and can be seen in government policy (Department of Health, 2009) and also in contemporary literature (Rath &

Harter, 2010; Seligman, 2011). As he says in his interview, one of his key well-being tools is '*the power of slow*'. Indeed, he calls this his '*golden tool*'.

Linden Lynn wrote some notes during his presentation at our psychosis conference, and I have drawn partly from these below. Augusto said, '*We cannot control the waves, but we can learn to surf the waves*'. He talked about his '*wellness toolbox*'. He stressed the need for partnership, both with loved ones and with professionals. He also talked about the need to accept loss, whatever form the loss might take in the individual sufferer's life. He highlighted the importance of self-knowledge, '*know thyself*'. This is also linked to being able to identify early warning signs of being unwell. He mentioned being in awe of and appreciating the wonder of ordinary things in life and in our own existence. '*Life is a climb*' he pointed out, '*but the view is great*'. Augusto draws on ancient Greek traditions to make points about hope and self-knowledge. A more contemporary Greek poet, Odysseus Elytis, expresses it thus, '*What I know not glows within me, and yet it glows*' (1996). It certainly glows brightly in Augusto.

Conclusion

Augusto stresses the importance of personal resilience. '*If I fall 1,000 times, then I will get up 1,000 times.*' He also talks about the importance of each individual asking themselves two key questions. '*Who am I now?*' '*What is it I want to accomplish from where I stand today?*'

References

Deegan P (1996) Recovery as a journey of the heart. *Psychiatric Rehabilitation Journal* **19** (3) 91–97.

Department of Health (2009) *New Horizons: A shared vision for mental health*. London: Department of Health.

Odysseus Elytis (1996) *The Oxopetra Elegies*. Amsterdam: Harwood Academic Publishers.

Rath T & Harter J (2010) *Wellbeing: The five essential elements*. New York: Gallup Press.

Seligman M (2011) *Flourish: A new understanding of happiness and wellbeing and how to achieve them*. London: Nicholas Brealey.

Further resources

Mind and Wellbeing Foundation [online]. Available at: www.mindandwellbeing.co.uk (accessed July 2011). Augusto D Mello is a consultant on the field of promoting healthy minds and co-founder of the Mind and Wellbeing Foundation.

Chapter 20

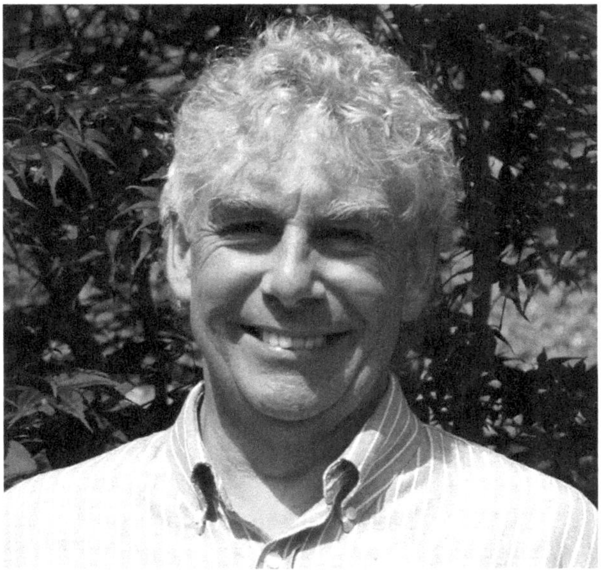

Glenn Roberts

Summary

Glenn trained as a psychiatrist, despite having quite a troubled childhood and in this chapter he describes his upbringing and that of his parents. Through psychiatry he found a 'kinship' with people in distress, and his own personal struggles with depression preceded his involvement with the recovery approach. Now retired, he still works part-time in the pioneering recovery service that he helped co-found.

Glenn in his own words

I was initially quite wary about contributing to this book as I have major concerns about both 'heroes' and 'handbooks'. I tended to agree with Sebastian Faulks (2010) who in reviewing our traditional representation of heroes, concluded that their day was over – or at least in their '*all conquering*' form and we often set up heroes only to knock them down again. I also had reservations about contributing to a 'handbook' in that I see recovery as fundamentally a matter of personal discovery – and so maps, models and handbooks all have value but risk over-defining how things could or should be and, in their simplified expectations, risk confusing people embarking on their own uncertain journeys.

On thinking about this further, I saw that transitions inherent in personal recovery for many, perhaps most, involve courage, commitment and responsibility – a sort of everyman heroism, as ordinary people find sufficient hope to use their strengths and creativity to overcome their difficulties. I was happy to contribute to a book of such stories which aims to hold out a hand to others on the basis that, '*We are all much more simply human than otherwise*' (Sullivan cited in Barton Evans, 1996) and there is of course a companionable warmth to be found amongst those who could be heroes for me, people who uphold values that I aspire to live by, in my personal and professional life.

So where have I come from? Many would quite rightly see my life as having been very successful, with a lengthy career as a consultant psychiatrist, with local and national recognition for my work and rich opportunities to offer creative contributions. I'm financially secure and happily married with four fine children all finding their way in the world as adults. Psychiatry has been very good to me and I hope I've contributed something positive to the development and delivery of mental health services. But this outwards appearance, my public CV, goes hand in hand with what has sometimes been a very different internal experience.

The dissonance between this outer and inner life troubled me deeply for many years but with maturity has come a growing reconciliation and narrowing of the gap. Now, in my mid 50s it seems that the abrasion, heat and struggle on the interface, has been the inspiration and motivation for much of what I've done and been able to achieve.

I was born in 1955 in East London to parents from poor and struggling backgrounds. My mother was one of eight children from the tenement district of Glasgow, Easterhouse, who were abandoned by their father, and she migrated to London to seek work and avoid bombs. My father was a Londoner and he lived at the school he attended where his father was the janitor, and where he died of a brain tumour when my father was 15. This left him studying alongside stoking the school boilers in order to avoid him becoming homeless.

My parents both struggled, but rather heroically my father got himself educated through night school and the army and eventually ended up owning a leading architect firm in WC1 in central London. They met on the dance floor; and I was named Glenn after their favourite bandleader, Glenn Miller. They had jumped many social and class divides within one generation but they experienced difficulties; my early life seemed full of tension, dispute and argument. I was unhappy and often difficult, truanting school and getting into fights, which I mostly lost. I was identified as an 'uncontrollable' or a 'disturbed child' and was nearly sent away to a remedial school – only my terror and pleading kept me at home, but I felt as though I was on probation for the rest of my childhood and I developed a lifelong fear of abandonment.

I don't know when I first experienced episodes of depression. As a young person I was aware that periodically I just ground to a halt, I couldn't think and didn't want to do anything. I withdrew and waited which I thought of as some kind of 'hibernation'. Later I became aware of an enduring sense of loneliness and disconnection from others, on top of which I have had times of profound sadness and occasionally despair. I somehow managed to live alongside this and developed an ambition to be a doctor. As with my father, this seemed an unlikely trajectory from where I'd come but I made it to medical school and continued to live a double life of outward successes and inward struggles with a sense of being a failure and misfit regardless of my actual achievements.

Looking back, I think my personal recovery began nearly 35 years ago, when at medical school I was first introduced to psychiatry and I found an inarticulate sense of kinship with people in deep distress. I had a fascination with learning about the intricacies of the mind and the puzzle of relationships. My personal landmarks included professional qualification and appointment as a consultant psychiatrist and moving with my family to a farmhouse and several acres in Devon in 1990. They also include the breakdown and loss of much of that, eight years later, in the context of my ongoing episodes of depression and the difficulty of sustaining my marriage. This led me to the worst period in my adult life in which I seriously considered dying, but in retrospect it was a 'low turning point' and the beginning of all that's been possible since.

Finding a happy and secure personal relationship has been the foundation for so much else, discovering 'recovery' from around the late 1990s onwards has been the most valuable, hopeful and creative discovery of my professional lifetime. My awareness of the recovery movement began with reading the personal and emancipation stories of people who had succeeded in their battle for recovery, often in very poor service settings. This inspired me to work for recovery within my profession and local services and at dismantling the stigmatising divide between 'them and us' in creative collaborations with people who use services. It has provided me with a conceptual compass, a guiding hope and a personal ambition which has kept me going ever since.

Glenn interviewed by Sophie

Glenn Roberts trained as a doctor in Bristol and worked for 30 years as a psychiatrist. Deeply interested in rehabilitation and concepts of recovery, he led on recovery for the Royal College of Psychiatrists and was co-founder of Recovery Devon, among a host of other activities. He has more than 60 publications to his name on a wide range of topics associated with recovery and psychosis. He was the Senior Editor of the award-winning *Enabling Recovery: The principles and practice of rehabilitation psychiatry* (Roberts *et al*, 2006). From his early years as a psychiatrist, Glenn was not happy with the idea of using drugs alone to treat mental illness. It was his belief that a unitary approach is not the most effective approach to what are often very complex problems. '*A whole range of issues and surrounding circumstances can play into mental illness. Someone might have depression but it could actually be about poverty. You need to take a whole life perspective,*' he commented.

Glenn has always struggled with the idea that psychiatrists defer to the so-called 'medical model', something which is portrayed with frequency in films and on television as the fundamentals of a psychiatrist's practice. This 'medical model' typically involves a restricted conceptualisation of mental illness as being the result of malfunctioning brains. It uses biological remedies i.e. drugs to 'correct' these malfunctioning brains and falls very short of picturing mental health problems as happening to people with a history in a context.

This narrow portrayal of the profession undermines and stigmatises medical practice as it is invariably seen to act as an impediment to recovery, according to Glenn. In all his years in the profession Glenn has never met a practitioner who exclusively subscribes to such a model and he believes that this skewed view of the profession is not useful and, moreover, serves to disconnect the profession as it is now from its origins.

Glenn's realisation that a '*whole-life*' or holistic approach is required in the face of mental illness led him into working in rehabilitation. Rehabilitation can be defined as '*regaining a life that you value and is satisfactory from your own point of view,*' said Glenn. It is no coincidence that all the major professional contributors to the recovery movement have migrated there from rehabilitation, he added.

For Glenn, the recovery approach is essentially a set of values incorporating, for instance, respect, equality, social inclusion, choice, and empowerment. This converts into a range of practices which are still being worked out. There is no fully worked out practice within recovery yet but lots of efforts in trusts all over the country to work it out.

In essence, the recovery approach is broader than individual treatment and could involve creativity, care of animals, gardening, or any other activity that somebody personally feels will aid their recovery. '*Personal stories of recovery are peppered with all sorts of things that don't fit into "evidence-based" treatment guidelines. The best thing is to work with people and enable them to find their own programme of recovery building on what they value, choose and experience to be useful,*' says Glenn.

It is a major step when people find the initiative to develop their own self-management. Mental illness is a spectrum, according to Glenn. At one end, people are very unwell and may find it extremely hard to stay safe and care for themselves. They will still require a large amount of input from skilled services and well-trained practitioners. At the opposite end of the spectrum, if perhaps mental health problems are identified early, people may find they can cope well with minimal professional help. In the middle ground, there are those people who can learn to self-manage with guidance and support from professionals and peers. '*You see a really major change when people become committed to their own recovery and also practitioners become so much more useful at this stage,'* said Glenn. All round, the environment for both practitioner and service user becomes hugely more positive when this happens, he added.

But also a practitioner has to sometimes face the uncomfortable reality that people can be deeper 'down the hole' of mental illness and therefore may find it harder to manage their recovery. Even in the deepest hole, however, the project remains one of enabling people to make their own decisions and take control of their own lives again. *'This gives recovery an educational emphasis, encouraging people to learn from their past and present experience and is a very different approach to one focused on treatment and what we do and for people,'* said Glenn.

The growth of the psychiatrist on a personal level is something which has long been an interest of Glenn's. *'You grow and mature yourself through work as a psychiatrist. Indeed this is one of the opportunities of this kind of work. You necessarily have to think deeply about who you are and what you're about. Of course this can represent a challenge but equally it is an opportunity to make sense of yourself.'*

As a trainee, Glenn was able to spend time with Dr Glin Bennet whose interest in the Jungian concept of the 'wounded healer' introduced him to ideas about the practitioner using his or her own personal struggles usefully to help someone heal rather than considering their own struggles as disqualifications. This naturally led him onto thinking about the health needs of the practitioners themselves. His interest in the narrative foundation of the practitioner's identity also dates back to these early beginnings, informed from digging into the histories of the founding fathers of psychiatry, some of whom were spiritual guides or dreamers. The idea therefore of a psychiatrist as a humanised healer who has also to work through his or her own struggles, and can then pass on their own knowledge and wisdom to another, is an attractive one to Glenn. Necessarily this kind of 'real life' acquired wisdom goes above and beyond the kind of knowledge gained purely through qualifications and underlines the need for practitioners to be selected and trained to develop their personal qualities too.

Glenn has now retired from his day job but continues to work one day a week in the Devon NHS Trust in the area of innovation and research. He leads a group who are supporting around 20 or so projects at present. He is also planning a two-day Autumn Festival of Recovery Innovations for people in Devon and recently led his trust's successful application to become a recovery practice development site under the NHS Confederation's programme Implementing Recovery: Organisational Change (ImROC). Excited as he is by these new projects, he is also keen to take up some of the more leisurely activities like fishing that retirement can allow him.

An appraisal of Glenn by Jerome

I was aware of Glenn's work on recovery before I started corresponding with him. The paper he co-authored with Dr Paul Wolfson was and still is a classic in the development of the recovery approach (Roberts & Wolfson, 2004). We had been in email contact for three years before eventually meeting up at the Refocus on Recovery Conference in London, in September 2010. Glenn was also a speaker at a one-day conference at the Institute of Psychiatry in February 2011, which I co-hosted.

Glenn's contribution to recovery is well known. What is less well known are his own personal struggles with depression. He described these in the book *Beyond the Storms*. He comments, *'At my lowest I sat up three days and nights weighing up whether to hang myself from a noose I'd set up for a hanging basket from a skylight. It would undoubtedly have worked,'* (Roberts, 2009). Thankfully, Glenn chose to live and went on to become one of the leading proponents of the recovery approach in Britain. He is the lead advisor on recovery to the Royal College of Psychiatrists. Along with other colleagues and service users in Devon, Glenn has done much to help inform, educate and inspire others. The Devon group has set up a really helpful recovery website (see www.recoverydevon.co.uk).

Glenn has also found inspiration in the work of New Zealand-based psychologist, Julie Leibrich. Her anthology of service user narratives has inspired many (Leibrich, 1999). Along with Jeremy Holmes, Glenn has also written a book on the importance of narrative in psychiatry (Roberts & Holmes, 1999) as well as several papers (Roberts, 2000; Roberts, 2011a). Glenn has stated that recovery is hard work (Roberts, 2011b). He knows that not just from his professional but also from his personal experience.

Conclusion

Glenn Roberts has worked as a psychiatrist for over 30 years. In the late 1990s he became aware of the recovery approach, which was developing around the world. He embraced this new approach and indeed became one of its leading exponents in Britain. His own experiences with depression have helped inform his narrative approach. While Glenn has now retired from full-time clinical work, this is unlikely to diminish his enthusiasm for recovery work.

References

Barton Evans F (1996) *Harry Stack Sullivan: Interpersonal theory and psychotherapy*. London: Routledge.

Faulks S (2010) *Faulks on Fiction: Great British characters and the secret life of the novel*. London: BBC Books.

Leibrich J (Ed) (1999) *A Gift of Stories*. Dunedin: University of Otago Press.

Roberts G & Holmes J (1999) *Healing Stories: Narrative in psychiatry and psychotherapy*. Oxford: Oxford University Press. (This book is available as a free download from the resource library at www.recoverydevon.co.uk).

Roberts G (2000) Narrative and severe mental illness: what place do stories have in an evidence based world? *Advances in Psychiatric Treatment* (**6**) 432–441.

Roberts G (2009) *Beyond the Storms: Reflections on personal recovery in Devon*. Exeter: Recovery Devon.

Roberts G (2011a) *Recovery and personal narratives*. In: H Cordle, J Fragdley, J Carson, F Holloway & P Richards (Eds) *Psychosis: Stories of recovery and hope*. London: Quay Books.

Roberts G (2011b) *Recovery for Practitioners: Stories to live by*. In: G McManus & J Carson (Eds) *From Communism to Schizophrenia and Beyond: One man's long march to recovery*. London: Whiting and Birch (unpublished).

Roberts G & Wolfson (2004) The rediscovery of recovery: open to all? *Advances in Psychiatric Treatment* **10** 37–49.

Roberts G, Davenport S, Halloway F & Tattan T (Eds) (2006) *Enabling Recovery: The principles and practice of rehabilitation psychiatry*. London: Gaskell.

Chapter 21

Conclusion

Jerome Carson, Elizabeth Wakely, Sophie Davies and Sarah Morgan

Job done?

In our introductory chapter, we outlined two main aims for this book. The first was to show how our five major historical recovery figures could be considered mental health recovery heroes and how their mental illnesses, in various ways and for different reasons, enhanced the contribution they were able to make to the world and humankind. The second was to gather together narratives from contemporary mental health recovery heroes, which might inspire professionals working with people with long-term mental health problems, their carers, and most importantly service users themselves.

Historical recovery heroes

As we stated at the start of the book, we were inspired to look at our five historical recovery heroes, by the short paper produced for the Time to Change campaign by Campbell & Jones (2009). Their thesis was that if their 'fantastic five' were alive today, then the discrimination that exists towards people with mental health problems might have stopped them achieving what they did. The world, they argued, would have been a completely different place without their unique contributions. We did of course choose to study Isaac Newton for our fifth hero, rather than Marie Curie, due to the fact that Liz and myself had become quite intrigued by his mental health problems from our background reading on Churchill, Nightingale and Darwin, from accounts about Newton in Storr (1989) and Pickering (1974). Liz's own thesis was that the lives of the so-called 'fantastic five' were to some degree enhanced by their mental illnesses. This thesis shared something in common with George Pickering's notion of a creative malady (Pickering, 1974).

In the first chapter in this book we looked at Winston Churchill. We concluded that his own experiences of depression helped him to understand and sympathise with the nation during the war years to boost their morale and to offer them hope and inspiration. We also argued, as did Storr (1989) that it was the manic aspects of his illness that gave him his 'trump card'. In 1940, a leader of sober judgement might have concluded that Britain was doomed, and that we ought to sue for peace with Hitler.

Florence Nightingale was the subject of our second chapter. While she is known in the popular imagination for her work during the Crimean War, we argued that her more important work was completed on her return to England. Despite a prolonged period of illness that lasted almost three decades she produced over 200 reports, pamphlets and booklets, not just on nursing, but on a wide range of other topics, from statistics to philosophy. While Bostridge (2008) claimed she suffered with brucellosis, other researchers have suggested she may also have had bipolar disorder or PTSD.

Our third chapter looked at Charles Darwin. In 1842, he moved to Down in Kent and started to lead a reclusive life, rarely venturing far from his house and becoming increasingly unwell. He published his magnum opus, *On the Origin of Species by Natural Selection* in 1859. While Campbell and Jones had claimed he suffered with an anxiety disorder, the clinical picture was more complex. A number of alternative diagnoses have been offered to explain Darwin's illness ranging from Chagas' disease to systemic lactose intolerance. Hubble offered the opinion that there were benefits arising from his clinical condition: '*...Darwin by his psychoneurosis secretly and passionately nourished his genius; he was protected thus from painful and wasted contacts, escaped from any circumstances which interfered with his work, was rewarded by sleepless nights of suffering which stimulated his restless mind,*' (Hubble, 1943).

Darwin himself acknowledged the benefits of his situation, '*...I have had ample leisure from not having to earn my own bread. Even ill health, though it has annihilated several years of my life, has saved me from the distraction of society and amusement,*' (Darwin cited in Neve & Messenger, 2002).

In chapter four we looked at Abraham Lincoln. As we pointed out, he was the only one of our five heroes who had books written about his mental health problems (Burlingame, 1997; Shenk, 2006). There is no doubt that he suffered with a recurrent depressive illness from his mid 20s, and as pointed out earlier in the book, it was said that '*his melancholy dripped from him as he walked*' (Herndon quoted in Shenk, 2006). Yet, here is the paradox with all these great people, namely that, '*...illness can co-exist with marvellous well-being*' (Shenk, 2006). Shenk also points out that while Lincoln meets the American Psychiatric Association's Diagnostic and Statistical Manual's definition of depression, he also meets the American Surgeon General's definition of mental health. According to Shenk, this is '*the successful performance of mental function resulting in productive activities, fulfilling relationships with other people and the ability to adapt and change and cope with adversity,*' (2006). Burlingame goes even further in quoting a psychologist who said of Lincoln, '*Lincoln achieved a kind of balance ... that he had more psychological honesty than anyone since Christ,*' (1997). Hence the famous expression 'Honest Abe'.

The final chapter in the historical recovery heroes section is on Isaac Newton, and he was probably the most difficult individual to research as the records are so much older and in parts incomplete. We know for instance that he destroyed many documents before he died, (Westfall, 1993). Despite this, new material continues to be researched, such as Levenson's (2009) new book on Newton's relationship with the counterfeiters. Achieving any clarity on the exact nature of Newton's mental health problems is probably impossible although it has not stopped many individuals trying, with the most recent claims of Professor Simon Baron Cohen that Newton may have had Asperger's syndrome (James, 2003). It may have been personality factors rather than mental illness, which led to Newton avoiding socialising and devoting himself obsessively to his studies and experiments, although as pointed out in the chapter, he seems to have become more sociable later in life.

We hope that our portrayals of these five historical recovery heroes have inspired readers and as we suggest that in many ways their mental health problems can be seen as having been advantageous to their life's achievements.

Contemporary recovery heroes

Our second aim for this book has been to draw together narratives from contemporary mental health recovery heroes, which might inspire mental health professionals, carers and service users. We had already written a series of five papers on recovery heroes. We updated these five accounts and added another ten accounts. Nearly everyone we approached agreed to take part in the book, with only two people declining.

The first contemporary recovery hero in the book was Peter Chadwick.

Peter is at the time of writing now 64 and retired, yet he continues to write on the topic of psychosis. Indeed he is probably the single most prolific writer in the book. No one has dissected their own psychosis as much as Peter in the process opening up all his 'family secrets'. Peter concludes that for him psychosis was a positive process although he suggests that probably less than 10% of sufferers will see it this way.

Dolly Sen was our second contemporary hero. Like Peter, Dolly has written an exposé of her early life experiences, which she feels contributed to the development of her own psychosis. Her two books on her story thus far make poignant reading. Since we first interviewed her she has gone onto successfully complete a degree course in film and video, achieving a first class honours degree. She is now working as a peer trainer in the country's first recovery college. She has also been very active in trying to dispel myths about madness and has been interviewed by Ruby Wax amongst others and is featured in Michelle McNary's *Recovery* film, and is on the Health Talk Online schizophrenia pages.

In Chapter 8, Emma Harding talked of her psychotic breakdown at university and her slow journey of recovery. This led her to train as a clinical psychologist. While previously very active in the service user movement she has been a little bit more reticent about her public profile, now she works as a psychologist within a mental health service. Even more significant, she has just become a mother.

Margaret Muir in Chapter 9 was our fourth contemporary hero. Margaret has been a local hero in the Lambeth service and has been the mainstay of our recovery group. She has also presented at conferences and has developed a new set of skills as a photographer. She reminds us that all service users who have battled with major mental disorders are all recovery heroes.

Michelle McNary in Chapter 10 has battled with a schizo-affective disorder for many years. She hopes to be able to turn the story of her battle into a new film of her struggles called *Climbing Walls*. It was the difficulty she had in approaching her own story that led us to suggest that her first film should be about a small group of other service users and their recovery journeys. This film deserves to join many of the other excellent recovery teaching resources in the public domain. Let's hope she has a similar success with *Climbing Walls*.

Stuart Baker-Brown in Chapter 11 told us of his journeys to Nepal and his climbs to Everest Base Camp. His remarkable journey can be witnessed in his equally remarkable photographs. He has also featured in the two Time to Change anti-discrimination videos, which will also help break down stigma. Like Peter Chadwick, he feels his illness has been a blessing in many ways. He was also awarded a very prestigious Churchill Travel Fellowship to make his first trip to Nepal. Let us hope he has many more journeys ahead.

In Chapter 12, Rachel Perkins told us of her three psychiatric careers and she let us know about her fourth career, now she has retired from full-time work. Having been professionally qualified as a clinical psychologist she then developed a bipolar illness. Despite this, she has managed to have a full and successful career, especially championing the importance of work in recovery. Like so many other contributors to the contemporary recovery heroes section of the book, we suspect there is much more to come from Rachel.

Andrew Voyce is probably one of the few people in mental health services who is grateful to Mrs Thatcher. He feels indebted to her for helping drive the closure of the old asylums, and establish the new model of community care. Andrew had been a '*revolving door*' patient for many years but has really thrived in the community. Like many of the contributors to the book, he does a lot of teaching on mental health issues and is also doing his own bit to break down the stigma.

Matthew Ward in Chapter 14 is a reluctant recovery hero. His own life had been a '*roller coaster*' ride of inexplicable highs and lows until he was diagnosed with a bipolar disorder in his early 40s. He puts this down to his own skills as an actor as well as the ineptitude of some of the doctors that he saw. His acting skills have been a great asset in spreading the recovery message.

Gordon McManus in Chapter 15 made the journey from communist philosopher to recovery philosopher, via a long almost 15 year diversion into schizophrenia. Gordon argues that for services to become more recovery focused will require a paradigm shift. Like many people, he refers to the 15 years of illness as his '*lost years*'. His work over the last few years is helping make up for the so called lost years.

Rufus May in Chapter 16 is one of the best known clinical psychologists in Britain. Indeed, he may be one of the only publicly known clinical psychologists in Britain. Like Emma Harding, he experienced a 'schizophrenic' breakdown in his late teens. The psychiatrists diagnosed Rufus with schizophrenia but as his chapter shows he looks at the episode differently. Rufus has also been very active in promoting a positive recovery focused message and challenging stigma.

Chapter 17 sees Peter Bullimore describing his own history of madness. He too is not enamoured with the term schizophrenia. Indeed he says, '*labels are for bottles and cans not people*' (Bullimore, 2011). Peter is also very active in teaching and has conducted training courses all over the world.

Bose Dania in Chapter 18 tells of her early career in dancing and how she had her first breakdown in Austria. There then followed a whole series of admissions to hospital. Bose began to work through her experiences through the medium of poetry. Indeed there can be few people who have written a poem on the Care Programme Approach (CPA) though many would agree with its concluding stanza:

CPA, they promise me support
So why do I feel so alone
CPA, when do we see the follow-up?
(Dania, 2011)

In Chapter 19, Augusto D Mello talks of his '*wellness toolbox*' and his '*golden tool*', which is '*the power of slow*'. He also echoes Patricia Deegan (1996) who talks about society accommodating or widening its boundaries to cover people on the fringes, or as Augusto describes it, 'being plus'.

In the final chapter, Glenn Roberts tells us of his own '*dark night of the soul*' and in finding recovery for himself, he found recovery for others. Glenn went on from his own depressive episode to become a leader in the recovery movement in Britain. The Devon Recovery Network has become one of the leading centres in disseminating recovery ideas and resources.

All 15 of our heroes were interviewed by Sarah and Sophie except for the two who were interviewed by Hannah Cordle. Sarah had this to say about this process:

'*I would like to say that it was a privilege to interview such inspiring and remarkably strong minded people. Working on this book has really shown the multi-faceted ways in which people can recover and deal with the challenges in their lives and it was a shame to have to edit down such interesting stories to the word count of the chapters, but I hope the essence of their struggle, achievements and message remains.'*

Common themes emerging from the narratives

While each story told in this book is of course unique to the individual telling it, as is their way of dealing with their problems in their recovery journey and their attitude towards recovery itself, there are however some common themes.

1. Identity and mental illness

All our authors seem to agree that it is important not to be defined and restricted by a diagnosis of mental illness and to accept one's situation. Rachel Perkins talks of '*disability in terms of barriers to acceptance put up by society*'. The next step is to find one's own identity, even if it is sometimes a bit nebulous and you may not always believe in it, but that self-belief is important as is the maintenance of hope. With this acceptance and self-awareness comes self-empowerment and responsibility in the setting of goals in order to lead a '*meaningful life*' as according to Gordon McManus. These vary considerably in their definitions and methods of attainment. Some are intimate or personal such as Bose Dania's poems, Margaret Muir's photography and for Gordon McManus, his chess. For some these are more physically ambitious, for example Stuart Baker-Brown and Everest Base Camp, some achieved by recognition in the public arena (Matthew Ward, Dolly Sen and Michelle McNary) and others in working for others (Bose Dania's charity work, Glenn Roberts, Rufus May, Emma Harding, Rachel Perkins, Peter Bullimore, Andrew Voyce, Stuart Baker-Brown and Augusto D Mello), but all are valid and validated by their outcomes. It is also important not to set these goals too high because, most people are not lucky enough to meet all three of Rachel Perkin's criteria for recovery: having somewhere to live, a job to do and someone to love, though almost everyone spoke of the importance of family and friends. Again, some people were more reticent than others about wanting to share their problems/experiences with others. (Rufus May and Glenn Roberts were very positive about this, whereas Emma Harding and Bose Dania said talking about them with people suffering from mental illness gets them down).

2. Attitudes to treatment in the NHS

Some individuals were very critical because of their experiences (see especially Andrew Voyce and also Stuart Baker-Brown) and of psychiatrists saying they were '*doomed*' (as with Peter Bullimore). Others were grateful and indeed have chosen to work within the NHS (see Emma Harding's story), but also perceive the need to combat entrenched views and raise awareness in professionals and in the public (see Rufus May), with many (especially Andrew Voyce and Rachel Perkins), very much in favour of care in the community.

3. Attitudes towards medication

This was probably the most controversial and polarised topic. Some of our recovery heroes were very critical because of their own personal experiences with medication, especially Rufus May, Dolly Sen and Andrew Voyce. Rufus May's experiences have partly inspired him to become a leading advocate for non-drug based therapies. Stuart Baker-Brown is very clear that his own recovery was helped by the right medication. Glenn Roberts states that while drugs have a role to play, other factors are also critical. Matthew Ward states that without lithium, he would probably be dead.

4. Other approaches

Dolly Sen and Michelle McNary both stressed the benefits of cognitive behavioural therapy. Others have not found it so helpful. Rufus May feels it is too expert led and formal.

5. A holistic approach

Glenn Roberts, Rufus May and Dolly Sen talk about seeing the whole person and not just looking at an illness. Several of our recovery heroes stressed the importance of family and friends.

6. The importance of narrative

Many of our recovery heroes believe in a narrative approach such as Peter Chadwick, Peter Bullimore, Augusto D Mello, Andrew Voyce and Dolly Sen. Most were agreed on the importance of professionals listening to, and being sensitive towards the experiences of people before they became ill, not just during their illness. With this comes the usefulness of self-knowledge, as with Augusto D Mello, and in certain cases, self-analysis, such as with Peter Chadwick.

What does the study of recovery heroes tell us?

A first lesson would be that you can find recovery heroes in all mental health services. Our own initial series of five recovery heroes featured four from our community mental health team in south west Lambeth. This was only one of the three such teams that covered the whole of Lambeth. We could probably have written this book just from the people who make up this one service. All staff working in mental health need to recognise that they have equally heroic individuals within their own services. These individuals can not only inspire them but can also inspire other service users.

A second lesson is that recovery is hard work (Roberts, 2009). Looking at our 15 contemporary recovery heroes none could be said to have had an easy time in life – all have had to battle. Many have made serious suicide attempts or have come close to doing so. Indeed Peter Chadwick survived after he threw himself under an oncoming bus but that was only due to the amazing reflexes of the bus driver who managed to swerve minimising the impact of his injuries. Having survived, Peter like all the recovery heroes featured, went on to make a huge contribution to our understanding of the recovery processes.

A third lesson is that each individual has to find their own unique path to recovery. For Rufus May and Emma Harding it was through training and becoming clinical psychologists, several years after they had been ill. Stuart Baker-Brown felt he needed to do something epic to prove that he could still do something major, just to show it was still possible for someone diagnosed with schizophrenia to do so. His journey led him to Nepal.

The fourth lesson is that it is possible to recover despite suffering a traumatic upbringing. Dolly Sen's childhood was almost Dickensian in nature. Peter Bullimore suffered prolonged sexual abuse from his babysitter and Peter Chadwick was bullied.

The fifth lesson is that despite where you start in your life journey, your recovery may take you on a completely different route. Gordon McManus started off in life as a communist philosopher and revolutionary, yet he ended up writing about the recovery revolution in mental health services. Margaret Muir only discovered a passion and aptitude for photography in her 60s. Augusto D Mello started in advertising selling products, yet now he has ended up '*selling*' well-being. Bose Dania went from dance to poetry.

Finally, each individual has relied on others to help them along their journeys. Emma Harding was helped by a psychologist in the hospital she was admitted to during her psychotic breakdown (Harding, 2011) and later on in life by two other psychologists, one who gave her the first job in mental health and another who encouraged her to apply for clinical training. Rufus May talked of being helped by a number of friends, who tolerated his somewhat unusual behaviour, without contacting the hospital as his family might have done. Dolly Sen talks of being helped by her first publisher, Jason Pegler, who believed in her. Sometimes, these people have been professionals, sometimes they have been friends.

Why are recovery heroes important?

We suggested in the introduction to the book that the notion of heroes is something that is culturally and historically important. In Britain at the moment there has been a campaign to try and bring attention to the work of the armed forces in conflict zones across the world, which is called Action for Heroes.

If we are to have a paradigm shift in mental health services we need to change the perceptions about people who use mental health services. There is considerable scepticism amongst many staff about the concept of recovery. The achievements of our contemporary recovery heroes can help counteract that scepticism. When Peter Chadwick came to speak about positive perspectives in psychosis at our local community team base in June 2009, we had 50 people present to hear him. Of the 50 people present, 25 were staff including one consultant psychiatrist. When Peter talked about his own personal recovery people were able to see the extent of the success he had achieved. Here was a man who despite suffering with a psychosis managed to obtain six degrees including PhDs in Geology and Psychology and a Doctor of Science degree for his research. A member of the audience suggested he could not be considered to be fully recovered as he was still taking medication. Peter conceded that he still took a small daily dose of haloperidol, but he asked the questioner if he thought he looked well. Peter pointed out that while this was a small dose it was part of what kept him well.

Every field of human endeavour needs its own heroes as role models. However, individuals need to be able to identify with heroes who share some of their own characteristics. Of the 15 contemporary heroes in this book, some have had no tertiary education. Some have come from minority communities where in addition to experiencing the effects of discrimination on mental health grounds they may also have experienced racism.

How does the concept of recovery heroes fit in with the concept of recovery?

The concept of recovery is best epitomised in the title of the Social Perspectives Network monograph, *Whose Recovery is it Anyway?* (2007). It is of course the service users' recovery. It follows therefore that we need to have an approach to recovery that places the experience of service users centre stage. Recovery heroes are individuals who are contributing to our developing understanding of what recovery is and how we can transform mental health services. In this book we have presented the stories of 15 recovery heroes and some of these have been actively involved in challenging the stigma associated with mental health by either taking part in films, or by appearing in the media. Others are trying to change the system from within through their work as mental health professionals. Some of our heroes are now accomplished trainers and try to inspire staff and other service users through their teaching role. Yet others are trying to develop our understanding of recovery processes through their writings. Again using creative skills of photography, poetry and acting are other ways that our heroes are getting across the message that recovery is possible. Recovery heroes can therefore be seen as being in the vanguard of the recovery approach. As Gordon McManus puts it, the goal of recovery is to help people cope with their symptoms of mental illness, but equally to help them develop more meaningful lives. We still have a long way to go on both fronts, yet the recovery heroes portrayed in this book, can help point the way forward.

References

Bostridge M (2008) *Florence Nightingale*. London: Penguin.

Bullimore P (2011) Forging his own destiny. In: H Cordle, J Fradgley, J Carson, F Holloway, F & Richards P (Eds) *Psychosis Stories of Recovery and Hope*. London: Quay Books.

Burlingame M (1997) *The Inner World of Abraham Lincoln*. Chicago: University of Illinois Press.

Campbell A & Jones N (2009) *A World Without: The fantastic five*. London: Time to Change.

Dania B (2011) *Life After Diagnosis* [online]. Available at: www.daniaspoetrycorner.co.uk (accessed July 2011).

Deegan P (1996) Recovery as a journey of the heart. *Psychiatric Rehabilitation Journal* **19** (3) 91–97.

Harding E (2011) A psychologists' progress. In: H Cordle, J Fradgley, J Carson, F Holloway, F & Richards P (Eds) *Psychosis Stories of Recovery and Hope*. London: Quay Books.

Hubble D (1943) Charles Darwin and psychotherapy. *The Lancet* 129–133.

James I (2003) Singular scientists. *Journal of the Royal Society of Medicine* (**96**) 36–39.

Levenson T (2009) *Newton and the Counterfeiters*. London: Faber.

Neve M & Messenger S (2002) *Charles Darwin – Autobiographies*. London: Penguin.

Pickering G (1974) *Creative Malady: Illness in the lives of Charles Darwin, Florence Nightingale, Mary Baker Eddy, Sigmund Freud, Marcel Proust and Elizabeth Barrett Browning*. London: George Allen and Unwin.

Roberts G (2009) Coming home. In: L Davidson, L Lynn (Eds) *Beyond the Storms: Reflections on mental health recovery in Devon*. Exeter: Devon Partnership NHS Trust.

Shenk J (2006) *Lincoln's Melancholy: How depression challenged a president and fuelled his greatness*. New York: Houghton Mifflin.

Social Perspectives Network (2007) *Whose Recovery is it Anyway?* London: Social Perspectives Network.

Storr A (1989) *Churchill's Black Dog and Other Phenomena of the Human Mind*. London: Harper Collins.

Westfall R (1993) *The Life of Isaac Newton*. Cambridge: Cambridge University Press.

BV - #0050 - 041218 - C0 - 246/189/14 - PB - 9781908066541